RENAL DIET FOOD LIST REFERENCE FOR KIDNEY DISEASE

Essential Foods and Recipes for Optimal Kidney Health

Dr. Thomas j. Millz

Copyright © 2024 [DR. THOMAS J. MILLZ]

All rights reserved. No part of this material may be reproduced, distributed, or transmitted in any form or by any means, including photocopying, recording, or other electronic or mechanical methods, without the prior written permission of the copyright owner, except in the case of brief quotations embodied in critical reviews and certain other noncommercial uses permitted by copyright law.

INTRODUCTION

Kidney infection is a difficult condition that influences a large number of individuals around the world. Proper nutrition plays a crucial role in managing this condition and improving quality of life. The kidneys are responsible for filtering waste and excess nutrients from the blood, and when they are not functioning properly, certain dietary adjustments become essential.

This book, "Renal Diet Food List Reference For Kidney Disease," is designed to help you understand which foods are beneficial and which should be limited or avoided. Whether you are a patient, caregiver, or healthcare professional, this guide aims to provide clear, practical information to support kidney health through diet.

You will find detailed food lists, sample meal plans, and recipes that cater to the specific needs of individuals with kidney disease. By following the guidelines in this book, you can make informed choices that will help manage your condition and improve your overall well-being.

Our Commitment

We are dedicated to providing accurate, up-to-date, and practical information to help you manage your kidney health through proper nutrition. Your wellbeing and prosperity are our main concerns, and we are here to help you constantly.

Together, let's take control of kidney disease with informed dietary choices and a commitment to a healthier future.

TABLE OF CONTENTS

INTRODUCTION..2
    1.1 Understanding Kidney Disease..4
    1.2 Importance of Diet in Kidney Health..8
    1.3 How to Use This Book...10

Basics of a Renal Diet..11
    2.1 What is a Renal Diet?...11
    2.2 Key Nutrients to Monitor..12
    2.2.1 Protein..12
    2.2.2 Sodium...14
    2.2.3 Potassium...16
    2.2.4 Phosphorus..18
    2.2.5 Fluids..20

Grocery Shopping for a Renal Diet..22
    3.1 Planning Your Shopping List...22
    3.2 Reading Food Labels..23
    3.3 Shopping Tips...24

Detailed Food Lists..26
    4.1 Fruits..26
    4.1.1 Low-Potassium Fruits...26
    4.1.2 High-Potassium Fruits to Avoid..28
    4.2 Vegetables...30
    4.2.1 Low-Potassium Vegetables..30
    4.2.2 High-Potassium Vegetables to Avoid...32
    4.3 Grains and Starches...35
    4.3.1 Recommended Grains..35
    4.3.2 Grains to Limit or Avoid..37
    4.4 Protein Sources..40

    4.4.1 Animal Proteins..40

    4.4.2 Plant-Based Proteins...43

    4.4.3 Protein Serving Sizes..46

    4.5 Dairy and Alternatives..48

    4.5.1 Low-Phosphorus Dairy Options..48

    4.5.2 Non-Dairy Alternatives..50

    4.6 Fats and Oils...53

    4.6.1 Healthy Fat Choices...53

    4.6.2 Fats to Avoid..56

    4.7 Beverages..59

    4.7.1 Hydration Tips...59

    4.7.2 Drinks to Limit or Avoid..62

    4.8 Snacks and Sweets..65

    4.8.1 Kidney-Friendly Snacks...65

    4.8.2 Sweets and Desserts...68

    4.9 Condiments and Seasonings..71

    4.9.1 Low-Sodium Options..71

    4.9.2 Herbs and Spices...74

Sample Menus and Meal Plans..77

    5.1 Weekly Meal Plan..77

    5.2 Exercises for kidney friendly patient..80

Renal Diet Recipes..83

    6.1 Breakfast...84

    6.2 Lunch..90

    6.3 Dinner...96

    6.4 Snacks...102

    6.5 Desserts..106

Managing Special Dietary Needs..111

    7.1 Diabetes and Kidney Disease..111

    7.2 Hypertension and Kidney Disease...112

    7.3 Vegetarian/Vegan Renal Diet 112

Living with a Renal Diet 114

    8.1 Dining Out Tips 115

    8.2 Traveling with a Renal Diet 115

    8.3 Coping with Dietary Changes 116

1.1 Understanding Kidney Disease

Kidney disease, also known as renal disease, encompasses a variety of conditions that impair the function of the kidneys. The kidneys are two bean-formed organs situated on one or the other side of the spine, just underneath the rib confine. Their primary function is to filter waste products and excess fluids from the blood, which are then excreted in the urine. The kidneys also play a crucial role in regulating blood pressure, maintaining electrolyte balance, and producing hormones that influence red blood cell production and bone health.

Types of Kidney Disease

1. **Chronic Kidney Disease (CKD):**
   - CKD is a drawn out condition described by a continuous loss of kidney capability over the long run. It is often caused by diabetes, high blood pressure, or other underlying health conditions. CKD is classified into five stages, with Stage 1 being the mildest and Stage 5 indicating kidney failure, which requires dialysis or a kidney transplant.
2. **Acute Kidney Injury (AKI):**
   - AKI is a sudden and often temporary loss of kidney function, usually due to an injury, infection, or a severe drop in blood flow to the kidneys. It can be caused by factors such as dehydration, severe infections, or complications from surgery.
3. **Glomerulonephritis:**
   - This condition involves inflammation of the glomeruli, which are tiny filtering units within the kidneys. It can be caused by infections, autoimmune diseases, or other conditions that affect the immune system.

4. **Polycystic Kidney Disease (PKD):**
   - PKD is a hereditary problem described by the development of various pimples in the kidneys. These cysts can enlarge the kidneys and impair their function over time.
5. **Kidney Stones:**
   - Kidney stones are hard stores of minerals and salts that structure inside the kidneys. They can cause severe pain and potential complications if not managed properly.

Symptoms of Kidney Disease

Kidney sickness frequently advances gradually and may not cause observable side effects in the beginning phases. Nonetheless, as the infection progresses, side effects might incorporate:

- Fatigue and weakness
- Swelling in the legs, ankles, or feet (edema)
- Shortness of breath
- Nausea and vomiting
- Persistent itching
- Changes in urine output and appearance
- Muscle cramps and twitches
- High blood pressure

Diagnosis and Treatment

Diagnosis of kidney disease typically involves blood tests to measure levels of creatinine and urea, which are waste products filtered by the kidneys. Urine tests can also help detect abnormalities such as protein or blood in the urine. Imaging tests, such as ultrasound or CT scans, and kidney biopsies may be used to assess the extent of kidney damage and identify underlying causes.

Treatment for kidney disease depends on the underlying cause and the stage of the disease. In early stages, lifestyle changes, including dietary modifications, managing blood pressure, and controlling blood sugar levels, can help slow the progression of the disease. Drugs might be recommended to oversee side effects and entanglements. In cutting edge stages, dialysis or a kidney relocate might be essential.

Understanding kidney disease is the first step in managing it effectively. By being informed about the condition, its symptoms, and treatment options, you can take proactive steps to protect your kidney health and improve your overall quality of life.

1.2 Importance of Diet in Kidney Health

Diet plays a critical role in managing kidney health and can significantly influence the progression of kidney disease. The kidneys are responsible for filtering waste and excess nutrients from the blood, and when they are compromised, dietary adjustments become essential to reduce the workload on these vital organs and maintain overall well-being.

Key Reasons Why Diet Matters

1. **Reducing Kidney Workload:**
   - A well-balanced diet tailored to kidney health can help reduce the strain on the kidneys. By managing the intake of certain nutrients such as protein, sodium, potassium, and phosphorus, you can lessen the kidneys' burden of processing and excreting these substances.

2. **Controlling Blood Pressure:**
   - Hypertension is both a reason and an outcome of kidney infection. A diet low in sodium and high in fruits and vegetables can help manage blood pressure levels and prevent further kidney damage. Reducing sodium intake helps decrease fluid retention and lowers blood pressure, which is crucial for kidney health.

3. **Managing Fluid Balance:**
   - In kidney disease, fluid balance becomes crucial. Excess fluid can lead to swelling, high blood pressure, and strain on the heart. A renal diet helps regulate fluid intake and minimizes the risk of fluid overload, which is especially important for individuals with advanced kidney disease.

4. **Controlling Blood Sugar Levels:**
   - For individuals with diabetes-related kidney disease, managing blood sugar levels is vital. A diet rich in low-glycemic index foods can help stabilize blood sugar levels and prevent complications related to diabetes and kidney health.

5. **Preventing or Managing Complications:**
   - Kidney disease often leads to complications such as anemia, bone disease, and cardiovascular issues. Diet can play a role in preventing or managing these complications. For example, adequate iron and vitamin D intake can help manage anemia and bone health.

6. **Maintaining Nutritional Balance:**
   - While managing specific nutrients, it's essential to ensure overall nutritional balance. A renal diet should provide sufficient energy, vitamins, and minerals to support general health without overloading the kidneys with harmful substances.

A carefully planned diet is a cornerstone of managing kidney disease and maintaining overall health. By adhering to dietary guidelines and making informed food choices, individuals with kidney disease can alleviate symptoms, slow disease progression, and improve their quality of life. Regular consultations with healthcare providers, including dietitians, can help tailor dietary recommendations to individual needs and ensure effective management of kidney health.

1.3 How to Use This Book

This book is designed to be a practical and accessible guide for managing kidney health through diet. Here's how to make the most of it:

1. **Refer to Detailed Food Lists:**
   - Use the comprehensive food lists to identify which foods are beneficial and which should be limited or avoided. This will help you make informed choices at the grocery store and when preparing meals.
2. **Utilize Sample Menus and Meal Plans:**
   - Follow the sample menus and meal plans for daily and weekly guidance on creating balanced, kidney-friendly meals. Adjust these plans based on your specific dietary needs and preferences.
3. **Explore Renal Diet Recipes:**
   - Try the recipes provided for breakfast, lunch, dinner, snacks, and desserts. Each recipe is designed to support kidney health while offering variety and flavor.
4. **Apply Special Dietary Guidelines:**
   - If you have additional health conditions such as diabetes or hypertension, refer to the sections on managing special dietary needs for tailored advice.
5. **Use Supplemental Information:**
   - Access the FAQs, glossary, and resource directory for additional support and information. These sections will help clarify any questions and guide you to further resources.

By following these guidelines, you can effectively navigate your dietary needs and make positive changes to support your kidney health.

Basics of a Renal Diet

2.1 What is a Renal Diet?

A renal diet is a specialized dietary plan designed to support kidney function and manage kidney disease. It focuses on controlling the intake of specific nutrients that the kidneys have difficulty processing, such as protein, sodium, potassium, and phosphorus. The primary goals of a renal diet are to reduce the kidneys' workload, manage fluid balance, and prevent complications associated with kidney disease. By following a renal diet, individuals can help slow the progression of kidney disease, maintain overall health, and improve quality of life.

2.2 Key Nutrients to Monitor

2.2.1 Protein

Protein is a fundamental supplement that assumes an urgent part in building and fixing tissues, delivering compounds and chemicals, and supporting general physical processes. In any case, for people with kidney illness, overseeing protein admission is especially significant.

Why Protein Matters in Kidney Health

1. **Kidney Function and Protein Processing:**
   o Healthy kidneys filter waste products from the blood, including those produced from protein metabolism. When kidney function is impaired, excessive protein can increase the strain on the kidneys, leading to further damage and complications.
2. **Balancing Protein Intake:**
   o A renal diet typically involves moderating protein intake to reduce the kidneys' workload while still meeting the body's nutritional needs. This balance helps minimize the buildup of waste products in the blood and reduces the risk of complications such as uremia.
3. **Quality of Protein:**
   o The focus is on consuming high-quality proteins that provide all essential amino acids. High-quality proteins include those from animal sources like lean meats, poultry, fish, and eggs, as well as some plant-based sources like soy products. These proteins are more efficiently used by the body and produce fewer waste products.

Recommendations for Protein Intake

- **Moderation:**
  - The amount of protein needed varies depending on the stage of kidney disease and individual health conditions. Generally, individuals with kidney disease are advised to consume lower amounts of protein compared to those with healthy kidneys. Specific recommendations should be provided by a healthcare professional or dietitian based on individual needs.

- **Portion Control:**
  - Proper portion sizes of protein-rich foods help manage intake levels. Measuring portions and tracking daily protein consumption can help ensure adherence to dietary guidelines.

- **Dietary Sources:**
  - Integrate an assortment of great protein sources into your eating regimen. Opt for lean meats, poultry, fish, eggs, and plant-based proteins like tofu and tempeh. Avoid excessive intake of processed meats and high-fat protein sources.

By carefully managing protein intake and focusing on high-quality sources, individuals with kidney disease can support their kidney health, prevent further damage, and maintain overall well-being.

2.2.2 Sodium

Sodium is a mineral that plays a crucial role in regulating fluid balance, blood pressure, and nerve function. However, excessive sodium intake can have significant impacts on kidney health, particularly for individuals with kidney disease.

Why Sodium Matters in Kidney Health

1. **Fluid Retention:**
   - Sodium helps regulate the body's fluid balance. When the kidneys are not functioning properly, they struggle to excrete excess sodium, leading to fluid retention. This can result in swelling (edema) in the legs, ankles, and feet, and can contribute to high blood pressure.
2. **Blood Pressure Control:**
   - High sodium intake is associated with elevated blood pressure, which can further damage the kidneys and increase the risk of cardiovascular complications. Managing sodium intake is crucial for controlling blood pressure and reducing strain on the kidneys.
3. **Impact on Kidney Function:**
   - Excess sodium can worsen kidney function by increasing the workload on the kidneys. By limiting sodium intake, individuals can help reduce kidney damage and manage symptoms more effectively.

Recommendations for Sodium Intake

- **Limit Sodium Consumption:**
  - The general recommendation for sodium intake is to consume less than 2,300 milligrams per day. For individuals with kidney disease, particularly those in advanced stages, the recommended limit may be even lower, often around 1,500 milligrams per day. Specific recommendations should be tailored by a healthcare provider or dietitian based on individual needs.

- **Read Food Labels:**
  - To manage sodium intake effectively, it's essential to read food labels carefully. Look for products labeled as "low sodium" or "no added salt," and avoid those with high sodium content. Processed and packaged foods, including canned soups, frozen meals, and snack foods, are often high in sodium.
- **Use Alternative Seasonings:**
  - Instead of salt, use herbs, spices, and other flavorings to enhance the taste of your meals. Options like garlic, lemon juice, and vinegar can add flavor without adding sodium.
- **Cook at Home:**
  - Getting ready feasts at home permits you to control how much sodium added to your food. Use fresh ingredients and cook from scratch whenever possible to reduce sodium intake.

By carefully managing sodium intake, individuals with kidney disease can help control blood pressure, reduce fluid retention, and minimize strain on the kidneys. This dietary adjustment is a key component of a renal diet and contributes to overall kidney health and well-being.

2.2.3 Potassium

Potassium is a vital mineral that helps regulate fluid balance, muscle contractions, and nerve function. It is also essential for maintaining healthy heart rhythms. However, for individuals with kidney disease, managing potassium intake is crucial, as impaired kidneys can struggle to maintain proper potassium levels in the body.

Why Potassium Matters in Kidney Health

1. **Kidney Function and Potassium Regulation:**
   - Healthy kidneys filter excess potassium from the blood. When kidney function is compromised, the body may retain excess potassium, leading to elevated blood potassium levels (hyperkalemia). High potassium levels can cause serious health issues, including irregular heartbeats and cardiac arrest.
2. **Risk of Hyperkalemia:**
   - Elevated potassium levels can have dangerous effects on the heart and overall health. Symptoms of hyperkalemia may include muscle weakness, fatigue, palpitations, and in severe cases, life-threatening arrhythmias.
3. **Impact of Diet:**
   - A diet high in potassium-rich foods can exacerbate hyperkalemia in individuals with kidney disease. Managing dietary potassium intake helps prevent complications and supports overall kidney function.

Recommendations for Potassium Intake

- **Monitor Potassium Consumption:**
  - The recommended potassium intake varies depending on the stage of kidney disease and individual health needs. Generally, individuals with kidney disease may need to limit their potassium intake to prevent hyperkalemia. A typical limit might range from 2,000 to 3,000 milligrams

per day, but specific recommendations should be provided by a healthcare professional.

- **Identify High-Potassium Foods:**
  - Foods high in potassium include bananas, oranges, potatoes, tomatoes, spinach, and certain nuts and seeds. Limiting these foods can help manage potassium levels. Select low-potassium choices and be aware of piece sizes.
- **Use Potassium-Reducing Techniques:**
  - Techniques such as soaking and leaching vegetables can reduce their potassium content. For instance, soaking potatoes in water for several hours and then boiling them can help lower their potassium levels.
- **Consult with a Dietitian:**
  - Working with a dietitian can provide personalized guidance on managing potassium intake. They can help create a balanced meal plan that meets your nutritional needs while controlling potassium levels.

By carefully managing potassium intake, individuals with kidney disease can help maintain safe potassium levels, reduce the risk of hyperkalemia, and support overall kidney health. Making informed dietary choices is essential for effectively managing kidney disease and enhancing quality of life.

2.2.4 Phosphorus

Phosphorus is a mineral that plays a key role in building and maintaining healthy bones and teeth, as well as in energy production and cellular function. However, for individuals with kidney disease, managing phosphorus intake is particularly important because impaired kidneys may struggle to regulate phosphorus levels effectively.

Why Phosphorus Matters in Kidney Health

1. **Kidney Function and Phosphorus Regulation:**
   - Healthy kidneys filter excess phosphorus from the blood. In kidney disease, the kidneys' ability to excrete phosphorus is diminished, leading to elevated phosphorus levels (hyperphosphatemia). High phosphorus levels can contribute to bone and cardiovascular problems.
2. **Impact on Bone Health:**
   - Elevated phosphorus levels can lead to a condition known as renal osteodystrophy, where bones become weakened and brittle. This is due to an imbalance of phosphorus and calcium in the body, which disrupts normal bone metabolism and can lead to bone pain and deformities.
3. **Cardiovascular Risks:**
   - High phosphorus levels can contribute to the development of cardiovascular issues, such as arterial calcification, which can increase the risk of heart disease.

Recommendations for Phosphorus Intake

- **Limit Phosphorus-Rich Foods:**
  - Many foods are high in phosphorus, including dairy products, nuts, seeds, meat, and processed foods. Limiting these foods can help manage phosphorus levels. Focus on consuming lower-phosphorus alternatives and be mindful of portion sizes.

- **Choose Phosphorus-Binders if Needed:**
    - In some cases, your healthcare provider may recommend phosphorus-binding medications that help reduce the absorption of phosphorus from food. These should be taken as prescribed and under the guidance of your healthcare provider.
- **Read Food Labels:**
    - Processed and packaged foods often contain added phosphorus in the form of phosphate additives. Reading food labels and choosing products with low or no added phosphorus can help control intake.
- **Work with a Dietitian:**
    - Collaborating with a dietitian can provide tailored guidance on managing phosphorus levels through diet. They can help create a meal plan that meets your nutritional needs while controlling phosphorus intake.

By managing phosphorus intake and making informed dietary choices, individuals with kidney disease can help maintain balanced phosphorus levels, support bone health, and reduce the risk of cardiovascular complications. Proper management of phosphorus is a critical aspect of a renal diet and contributes to overall kidney health.

2.2.5 Fluids

Fluids are essential for maintaining bodily functions such as digestion, circulation, and temperature regulation. However, for individuals with kidney disease, managing fluid intake is crucial as impaired kidneys may struggle to balance fluid levels effectively.

Why Fluid Management Matters in Kidney Health

1. **Fluid Retention:**
   - When the kidneys are not functioning properly, they may have difficulty excreting excess fluids from the body. This can lead to fluid retention, causing swelling (edema) in the legs, ankles, and other parts of the body, as well as potentially increasing blood pressure.
2. **Managing Blood Pressure:**
   - Excess fluid in the body can contribute to high blood pressure, which can further damage the kidneys and increase the risk of cardiovascular problems. Controlling fluid intake helps manage blood pressure and reduce strain on the kidneys.
3. **Preventing Fluid Overload:**
   - In advanced stages of kidney disease, fluid overload can lead to complications such as shortness of breath, congestive heart failure, and pulmonary edema. Proper fluid management is essential to prevent these complications.

Recommendations for Fluid Intake

- **Monitor Fluid Intake:**
  - The recommended fluid intake varies based on the stage of kidney disease and individual health needs. Your healthcare provider or dietitian will provide specific guidelines on how much fluid you should consume daily.

- **Track All Sources of Fluids:**
    - Fluid intake includes not only drinking water but also beverages like tea, coffee, and milk, as well as fluids in soups, sauces, and even fruits and vegetables with high water content. Be mindful of all sources when managing fluid intake.
- **Use Fluid Restriction Techniques:**
    - If fluid restriction is necessary, consider using measuring cups or bottles to track your fluid consumption. This can help you stay within your prescribed limits.
- **Manage Thirst:**
    - For some individuals, managing thirst can be challenging. Using strategies such as sucking on ice chips, chewing gum, or consuming small amounts of fluids throughout the day can help alleviate thirst while staying within fluid limits.
- **Consult with a Dietitian:**
    - A dietitian can provide personalized advice on fluid management and help create a plan that balances your hydration needs with your kidney health.

By carefully managing fluid intake and following the guidelines provided by healthcare professionals, individuals with kidney disease can help maintain a healthy fluid balance, manage blood pressure, and prevent complications associated with fluid overload. Fluid management is a critical component of a renal diet and contributes to overall kidney health and well-being.

Grocery Shopping for a Renal Diet

3.1 Planning Your Shopping List

Planning your shopping list is essential for maintaining a renal diet and managing kidney health effectively. Here's how to make it work:

1. **Prioritize Kidney-Friendly Foods:**
    - Focus on including low-sodium, low-potassium, and low-phosphorus options. Prioritize fresh fruits and vegetables, lean proteins, and whole grains that meet dietary guidelines.
2. **Read Labels Carefully:**
    - Choose products with minimal added sodium and phosphate additives. Look for labels that specify low-sodium or no added salt.
3. **Plan Balanced Meals:**
    - Create a list based on planned meals and snacks to ensure variety and balance. Include items that fit within your dietary restrictions and provide essential nutrients.
4. **Avoid Processed Foods:**
    - Minimize purchases of processed and packaged foods, which often contain high levels of sodium and phosphorus. Choose new, entire food sources whenever the situation allows.

By carefully planning your shopping list, you can stay on track with your renal diet, make healthier food choices, and better manage your kidney health.

3.2 Reading Food Labels

Reading food labels is crucial for managing a renal diet. Focus on the following:

1. **Check Sodium Content:**
   - Look for products with low or no added sodium. Aim for items with less than 140 milligrams of sodium per serving to help manage blood pressure and fluid retention.
2. **Identify Potassium and Phosphorus Levels:**
   - Some labels list potassium and phosphorus content. Choose foods with lower levels to avoid excess intake.
3. **Watch for Additives:**
   - Avoid products with phosphate additives, often listed as "phosphate" or "phosphoric acid," which can increase phosphorus levels.
4. **Review Serving Sizes:**
   - Pay attention to serving sizes to accurately gauge nutrient intake and ensure you're not consuming more than recommended.

By carefully examining food labels, you can make informed choices that align with your dietary needs and support kidney health.

3.3 Shopping Tips

Effective shopping is key to adhering to a renal diet. Here are some tips to make your grocery trips easier and healthier:

1. **Make a List:**
    - Create a detailed shopping list based on your meal plan and dietary needs. This helps avoid impulse buys and ensures you purchase only kidney-friendly foods.
2. **Shop the Perimeter:**
    - Center around the edge of the store, where new produce, lean meats, and dairy items are ordinarily found. Avoid the inner aisles where processed and high-sodium foods are often found.
3. **Choose Fresh Over Processed:**
    - Opt for fresh fruits, vegetables, and whole grains rather than processed foods, which often contain high levels of sodium, phosphorus, and additives.
4. **Use Frozen and Canned Wisely:**
    - If buying frozen or canned items, select those with no added salt or sugar. Rinse canned foods to reduce sodium content when possible.
5. **Check for Low-Sodium Options:**
    - Look for low-sodium or no-sodium-added versions of products like soups, sauces, and condiments to manage your intake more effectively.
6. **Read Labels Thoroughly:**
    - Always check food labels for sodium, potassium, and phosphorus content to ensure they fit within your dietary restrictions.
7. **Plan for Leftovers:**
    - Buy in quantities that align with your meal planning to minimize food waste and make meal preparation easier.

By following these shopping tips, you can better manage your renal diet, make healthier food choices, and support your kidney health effectively.

Detailed Food Lists

4.1 Fruits

4.1.1 Low-Potassium Fruits

Low-potassium fruits are an essential part of a renal diet, offering vital nutrients and natural sweetness without overwhelming the kidneys with excess potassium. Including these fruits in your diet can help maintain balanced potassium levels while still enjoying a variety of flavors and textures.

Common Low-Potassium Fruits

1. **Apples:**
   - Apples are versatile and can be eaten raw, baked, or added to salads. They are low in potassium and high in fiber, making them a healthy choice for kidney health.
2. **Berries:**
   - Strawberries, blueberries, raspberries, and blackberries are all low in potassium and rich in antioxidants, vitamins, and fiber. They can be enjoyed fresh, in smoothies, or as toppings for cereals and desserts.
3. **Grapes:**
   - Grapes are another low-potassium option that can be eaten fresh, frozen, or used in salads. They are likewise a decent wellspring of hydration because of their high water content.
4. **Peaches:**
   - Fresh peaches, particularly when eaten in moderation, are a low-potassium fruit that can be enjoyed on their own or as part of a fruit salad.

5. **Pineapple:**
   - Pineapple is a tropical fruit that is low in potassium and can add a burst of flavor to your meals. It can be eaten fresh, grilled, or used in salsas and desserts.
6. **Cranberries:**
   - Cranberries are not only low in potassium but also beneficial for urinary tract health. They can be consumed as juice (without added sugar), dried, or fresh.

Tips for Including Low-Potassium Fruits in Your Diet

- **Portion Control:**
  - Even low-potassium fruits should be consumed in appropriate portions to maintain balanced potassium levels. Aim for small servings throughout the day.
- **Variety:**
  - Incorporate a variety of low-potassium fruits into your diet to enjoy different flavors and nutritional benefits without exceeding potassium limits.
- **Use in Recipes:**
  - Add low-potassium fruits to smoothies, salads, yogurt, or as a snack. They can also be used to naturally sweeten baked goods.

By choosing low-potassium fruits, you can enjoy a nutrient-rich diet that supports kidney health while keeping potassium levels in check.

4.1.2 High-Potassium Fruits to Avoid

For individuals with kidney disease, managing potassium intake is crucial, as high potassium levels can lead to serious health complications. Certain fruits, while nutritious, are naturally high in potassium and should be limited or avoided to prevent the risk of hyperkalemia.

Common High-Potassium Fruits to Avoid

1. **Bananas:**
    - Bananas are well-known for their high potassium content. A single medium banana can contain over 400 milligrams of potassium, making them a fruit to avoid or strictly limit in a renal diet.
2. **Oranges and Orange Juice:**
    - Oranges and orange juice are rich in potassium, with one orange containing around 240 milligrams and a cup of orange juice containing even more. It's best to choose lower-potassium fruit alternatives.
3. **Avocados:**
    - While avocados are packed with healthy fats, they are also high in potassium. Half an avocado can contain around 500 milligrams of potassium, so it's recommended to avoid them in a kidney-friendly diet.
4. **Tomatoes and Tomato-Based Products:**
    - Tomatoes, including tomato sauce and tomato juice, are high in potassium. A single cup of tomato juice can contain over 600 milligrams of potassium, making it a fruit to avoid.
5. **Cantaloupe and Honeydew Melon:**
    - These melons are sweet and refreshing but also high in potassium. A small slice of cantaloupe or honeydew melon can contribute significantly to daily potassium intake.

6. **Dried Fruits:**
    - Dried fruits, such as raisins, apricots, and prunes, are concentrated sources of potassium. A small handful can easily exceed recommended potassium limits for those with kidney disease.
7. **Mangoes:**
    - Mangoes, while delicious, are also high in potassium, with one cup of sliced mango containing around 300 milligrams. It's best to limit or avoid them in a renal diet.

Tips for Managing High-Potassium Fruits

- **Portion Control:**
    - If you occasionally consume high-potassium fruits, keep portion sizes very small and factor them into your overall daily potassium intake.
- **Substitute with Low-Potassium Options:**
    - Replace high-potassium fruits with low-potassium alternatives like apples, berries, or grapes to still enjoy fruit without the excess potassium.
- **Consult with a Dietitian:**
    - Work with a dietitian to develop a meal plan that manages potassium levels effectively while still including a variety of fruits.

By avoiding or limiting high-potassium fruits, individuals with kidney disease can better manage their potassium levels and reduce the risk of complications associated with hyperkalemia. Making informed choices about fruit intake is an essential part of maintaining kidney health.

4.2 Vegetables

4.2.1 Low-Potassium Vegetables

Low-potassium vegetables are a vital component of a renal diet, providing essential vitamins, minerals, and fiber while keeping potassium levels in check. Incorporating these vegetables into your meals can help maintain kidney health without the risk of elevated potassium levels.

Common Low-Potassium Vegetables

1. **Cabbage:**
   - Cabbage is a versatile, low-potassium vegetable that can be eaten raw in salads, sautéed, or added to soups and stews. It is rich in vitamins C and K and provides a good source of fiber.

2. **Cauliflower:**
   - Cauliflower is another low-potassium vegetable that can be enjoyed roasted, mashed, or as a rice substitute. It's packed with vitamin C, folate, and fiber, making it a nutritious choice for a renal diet.

3. **Bell Peppers:**
   - Bell peppers, especially the green variety, are low in potassium and high in vitamins A and C. They add color, crunch, and nutrition to salads, stir-fries, and sandwiches.

4. **Lettuce:**
   - Lettuce, particularly iceberg and romaine, is low in potassium and can be used as a base for salads or in sandwiches. It provides hydration and is low in calories.

5. **Onions:**
   - Onions are low in potassium and can be used to add flavor to a wide variety of dishes. They are also rich in antioxidants and beneficial for heart health.

6. **Green Beans:**
   - Green beans are a low-potassium vegetable that can be steamed, sautéed, or added to casseroles. They are also a good source of fiber and vitamin C.
7. **Cucumbers:**
   - Cucumbers are hydrating and low in potassium, making them a refreshing addition to salads and sandwiches. They are likewise low in calories and give a decent wellspring of nutrients K and C.

Tips for Including Low-Potassium Vegetables in Your Diet

- **Variety:**
  - Incorporate a wide range of low-potassium vegetables into your meals to ensure you get a variety of nutrients. This helps keep meals interesting and nutritionally balanced.
- **Cooking Methods:**
  - Cooking methods like steaming, roasting, or boiling can enhance the flavor of low-potassium vegetables while maintaining their nutritional value. Avoid overcooking, as it can lead to nutrient loss.
- **Use in Recipes:**
  - Add low-potassium vegetables to salads, soups, stir-fries, or as side dishes. They can also be used as a base for casseroles and other main dishes.
- **Portion Control:**
  - Even with low-potassium vegetables, it's important to monitor portion sizes to ensure overall potassium intake remains within recommended limits.

By focusing on low-potassium vegetables, individuals with kidney disease can enjoy a nutritious and varied diet that supports their health while keeping potassium levels under control.

4.2.2 High-Potassium Vegetables to Avoid

Managing potassium intake is crucial for individuals with kidney disease, as high levels of potassium can lead to serious health complications. Certain vegetables, while nutritious, are naturally high in potassium and should be limited or avoided to prevent hyperkalemia.

Common High-Potassium Vegetables to Avoid

1. **Potatoes:**
   - Potatoes, including white, red, and sweet varieties, are high in potassium. A single medium potato can contain over 900 milligrams of potassium, making them a vegetable to limit or avoid in a renal diet. Techniques such as leaching (soaking in water before cooking) can reduce potassium content, but caution is still advised.

2. **Tomatoes:**
   - Tomatoes and tomato-based products, such as sauces, juices, and pastes, are rich in potassium. A cup of tomato sauce can contain over 800 milligrams of potassium, making it a high-potassium vegetable to steer clear of in large quantities.

3. **Spinach:**
   - Spinach is nutrient-dense but also high in potassium, particularly when cooked. One cup of cooked spinach can contain nearly 850 milligrams of potassium. Raw spinach has less, but portion control is still necessary.

4. **Avocados:**
   - Although often categorized as a fruit, avocados are frequently used in savory dishes and are high in potassium. Half an avocado can contribute around 500 milligrams of potassium, so it's best to avoid or strictly limit them.

5. **Beets:**
    - Beets, including beet greens, are high in potassium, with a single cup of cooked beets containing over 500 milligrams of potassium. Both the root and greens should be avoided or limited in a renal diet.
6. **Brussels Sprouts:**
    - Brussels sprouts, while healthy in many ways, are high in potassium. A cup of cooked Brussels sprouts can contain about 500 milligrams of potassium, making them a vegetable to consume in moderation.
7. **Artichokes:**
    - Artichokes are another high-potassium vegetable, with a medium artichoke containing around 400 milligrams of potassium. It's best to avoid them or eat them in very small portions.

Tips for Managing High-Potassium Vegetables

- **Portion Control:**
    - If you occasionally consume high-potassium vegetables, keep portion sizes small and be aware of your overall daily potassium intake.
- **Substitution:**
    - Replace high-potassium vegetables with lower-potassium alternatives such as cauliflower, green beans, or bell peppers to maintain variety without the excess potassium.
- **Preparation Techniques:**
    - Certain methods, like soaking potatoes or leaching other high-potassium vegetables, can reduce potassium content, but it's essential to consult with a dietitian before relying on these methods.
- **Consult with a Dietitian:**
    - A dietitian can provide guidance on managing potassium intake and suggest appropriate substitutes for high-potassium vegetables in your diet.

By avoiding or strictly limiting high-potassium vegetables, individuals with kidney disease can better manage their potassium levels and reduce the risk of complications associated with hyperkalemia. Making informed choices about vegetable intake is a key aspect of maintaining kidney health.

4.3 Grains and Starches

4.3.1 Recommended Grains

Grains are an important part of a balanced diet, providing essential carbohydrates, fiber, and nutrients. For individuals with kidney disease, choosing the right grains is crucial to managing phosphorus and potassium intake while still benefiting from the energy and nutrition that grains offer.

Common Recommended Grains

1. **White Rice:**
    - White rice is a low-potassium, low-phosphorus grain that is easy to digest and versatile in cooking. It can be used as a base for meals, in soups, or as a side dish, making it a staple in a renal diet.
2. **Refined Pasta:**
    - Refined pasta, made from white flour, is lower in potassium and phosphorus compared to whole-grain varieties. It can be used in a variety of dishes, including salads, soups, and main courses, offering a good source of energy.
3. **White Bread:**
    - White bread, made from refined flour, is lower in potassium and phosphorus compared to whole-grain bread. It can be included in meals as toast, sandwiches, or as an accompaniment to soups and salads.
4. **Cornmeal:**
    - Cornmeal is another low-potassium, low-phosphorus grain option that can be used to make polenta, cornbread, or as a coating for baked foods. It provides a good source of energy and can be easily incorporated into meals.

5. **Rice Cereal:**
   - Rice cereal, such as puffed rice or cream of rice, is a renal-friendly grain option for breakfast. It is low in potassium and phosphorus and can be enjoyed with low-potassium fruits or as a snack.
6. **Couscous:**
   - Couscous, made from semolina wheat, is a low-potassium grain that cooks quickly and can be used in salads, as a side dish, or in main courses. It is light and versatile, making it an excellent choice for a renal diet.

Tips for Including Recommended Grains in Your Diet

- **Focus on Refined Grains:**
  - While whole grains are typically more nutritious, they are also higher in potassium and phosphorus. For those with kidney disease, refined grains like white rice, white bread, and refined pasta are better choices to manage these nutrients.
- **Pair with Low-Potassium Foods:**
  - Combine grains with low-potassium vegetables and lean proteins to create balanced, kidney-friendly meals that support overall health.
- **Portion Control:**
  - Be mindful of portion sizes to ensure that your carbohydrate intake is balanced with other food groups, preventing excess calorie consumption.
- **Variety:**
  - Incorporate a variety of recommended grains into your diet to keep meals interesting and provide different textures and flavors.

By choosing the right grains, individuals with kidney disease can enjoy nutritious, energy-rich meals while effectively managing their potassium and phosphorus intake. These recommended grains are key to maintaining a balanced and renal-friendly diet.

4.3.2 Grains to Limit or Avoid

For individuals with kidney disease, certain grains may need to be limited or avoided due to their high content of potassium, phosphorus, or other nutrients that can place additional strain on the kidneys. Managing these grains carefully is essential to maintaining kidney health.

Common Grains to Limit or Avoid

1. **Whole Wheat Bread:**
    - Whole wheat bread is rich in fiber and nutrients, but it also contains higher levels of potassium and phosphorus compared to white bread. For those with kidney disease, it's advisable to limit its consumption or opt for white bread instead.
2. **Brown Rice:**
    - Brown rice, while more nutritious than white rice, contains significantly more potassium and phosphorus. A cup of cooked brown rice can contribute to an excessive intake of these minerals, making it a grain to avoid or limit.
3. **Oatmeal:**
    - Oatmeal is a healthy whole grain but is higher in phosphorus and potassium than many refined grains. While it can be consumed in small portions, it's important to monitor your overall daily intake of these minerals.
4. **Quinoa:**
    - Quinoa is a complete protein and a popular whole grain, but it is also high in potassium and phosphorus. It should be limited or avoided by those managing kidney disease to prevent excess intake of these nutrients.

5. **Bran Cereals:**
    - Bran cereals, including those made from wheat or oats, are high in both fiber and phosphorus. These cereals should be avoided or consumed in very limited amounts, as they can contribute to elevated phosphorus levels.
6. **Barley:**
    - Barley, though nutritious, is higher in potassium and phosphorus. It is best to limit its use in soups, salads, or as a grain side dish if you're following a renal diet.
7. **Whole Grain Pasta:**
    - Whole grain pasta, while richer in nutrients and fiber than refined pasta, also contains more potassium and phosphorus. It's recommended to choose refined pasta instead to keep potassium and phosphorus intake lower.

Tips for Managing High-Phosphorus and High-Potassium Grains

- **Portion Control:**
    - If consuming whole grains, keep portions small and be mindful of your overall daily intake of potassium and phosphorus.
- **Alternative Grains:**
    - Opt for lower-potassium and lower-phosphorus grains like white rice, refined pasta, or couscous. These options allow you to enjoy grains without exceeding nutrient limits.
- **Consult a Dietitian:**
    - Work with a dietitian to tailor your grain choices to your specific needs, ensuring you get the necessary nutrients without overloading on potassium or phosphorus.
- **Read Labels:**
    - When purchasing grains or grain-based products, carefully read labels to check for potassium and phosphorus content. Some products may have added phosphorus-based preservatives, which should be avoided.

By limiting or avoiding these high-potassium and high-phosphorus grains, individuals with kidney disease can better manage their nutrient intake and reduce the risk of complications associated with elevated potassium and phosphorus levels. Making informed choices about grain consumption is a key aspect of maintaining kidney health and supporting overall well-being

4.4 Protein Sources

4.4.1 Animal Proteins

Animal proteins are an important source of essential amino acids, which the body needs for tissue repair, muscle maintenance, and overall health. However, for individuals with kidney disease, it's important to manage the intake of animal proteins carefully to prevent overburdening the kidneys with waste products and excessive phosphorus.

Recommended Animal Proteins

1. **Chicken (Skinless):**
   - Skinless chicken is a lean source of protein that is lower in phosphorus compared to red meats. It can be baked, grilled, or poached to minimize added fats and maintain its renal-friendly profile.
2. **Turkey:**
   - Like chicken, turkey is a lean protein option that is lower in phosphorus and potassium. It's versatile and can be included in a variety of dishes, from sandwiches to salads.
3. **Fish (Low-Phosphorus Varieties):**
   - Certain fish, such as cod, sole, and tilapia, are lower in phosphorus and can be safely included in a renal diet. These fish are also rich in omega-3 fatty acids, which are beneficial for heart health.
4. **Egg Whites:**
   - Egg whites are an excellent source of high-quality protein without the added phosphorus found in egg yolks. They can be used in omelets, scrambled, or added to various recipes as a protein boost.
5. **Pork (Lean Cuts):**
   - Lean cuts of pork, such as tenderloin, are lower in phosphorus and can be consumed in moderation. Cooking methods like grilling or baking help keep pork a healthy option.

Animal Proteins to Limit or Avoid

1. **Red Meat (Beef, Lamb):**
   - Red meats are generally higher in phosphorus and potassium, and their regular consumption can strain the kidneys. If consumed, they should be limited to small portions and lean cuts.
2. **Processed Meats (Bacon, Sausages):**
   - Processed meats are often high in sodium, phosphorus, and other additives that are harmful to kidney health. These should be avoided or eaten very sparingly.
3. **Shellfish:**
   - Shellfish, including shrimp, crab, and lobster, are high in phosphorus and should be limited in a renal diet. They can contribute to elevated phosphorus levels, which can be harmful to the kidneys.
4. **Organ Meats (Liver, Kidney):**
   - Organ meats are rich in protein but also extremely high in phosphorus and other waste products. They should be avoided to prevent overloading the kidneys.
5. **Deli Meats:**
   - Deli meats, such as ham and turkey slices, are often high in sodium and phosphorus due to preservatives. Opt for fresh, unprocessed meats instead.

Tips for Including Animal Proteins in Your Diet

- **Portion Control:**
  - Keep portions small, typically around 3 ounces per serving, to manage protein intake without overloading the kidneys.
- **Cooking Methods:**
  - Choose cooking methods that don't add extra fats or sodium, such as grilling, baking, or steaming. Avoid frying and heavy sauces that can increase the burden on the kidneys.

- **Pair with Low-Potassium Foods:**
  - Balance animal proteins with low-potassium vegetables and grains to create meals that support kidney health.
- **Consult with a Dietitian:**
  - Work with a dietitian to determine the right amount and types of animal proteins for your specific needs, ensuring you get the essential nutrients without straining your kidneys.

By selecting the right types of animal proteins and managing portion sizes, individuals with kidney disease can enjoy the benefits of high-quality protein while protecting their kidney health. Making informed choices about animal proteins is crucial for maintaining a balanced and renal-friendly diet.

4.4.2 Plant-Based Proteins

Plant-based proteins are an important component of a kidney-friendly diet, offering essential nutrients without the high levels of phosphorus and saturated fat often found in animal proteins. For individuals with kidney disease, incorporating plant-based proteins can help meet protein needs while managing kidney health.

Recommended Plant-Based Proteins

1. **Tofu:**
   - Tofu, made from soybeans, is a versatile and low-phosphorus protein source. It can be used in a variety of dishes, from stir-fries to salads, and is an excellent substitute for meat.
2. **Tempeh:**
   - Tempeh is another soy-based protein that is fermented, making it easier to digest. It is higher in protein than tofu and can be grilled, sautéed, or added to stews and casseroles.
3. **Beans (in Moderation):**
   - While beans like kidney beans, black beans, and chickpeas are high in protein, they also contain moderate levels of potassium and phosphorus. It's important to consume them in moderation and monitor portion sizes.
4. **Lentils:**
   - Lentils are a good source of plant-based protein and fiber, but they also contain phosphorus. Small portions can be included in a renal diet, particularly when prepared with methods that reduce phosphorus content, such as soaking.
5. **Quinoa (in Moderation):**
   - Quinoa is a complete protein, meaning it contains all nine essential amino acids. While it is higher in phosphorus, it can be consumed in small portions as part of a balanced renal diet.

6. **Hemp Seeds:**
   - Hemp seeds are rich in protein and healthy fats, and they are lower in phosphorus compared to other seeds. They can be sprinkled on salads, added to smoothies, or used in baking.
7. **Peas:**
   - Peas, including green peas and split peas, provide a good source of protein and fiber. They are lower in phosphorus than beans and can be used in soups, salads, or as a side dish.

Plant-Based Proteins to Limit or Avoid

1. **Nuts:**
   - While nuts are high in protein, they also contain significant amounts of phosphorus and potassium. They should be limited in a renal diet, and lower-phosphorus nuts like macadamia nuts can be chosen in small amounts.
2. **Soy Products (High in Phosphorus):**
   - Some soy products, like soy milk and edamame, are higher in phosphorus and should be consumed in moderation or avoided, depending on your dietary needs.
3. **Seeds (Sunflower, Pumpkin):**
   - Seeds like sunflower and pumpkin seeds are high in phosphorus and should be limited in a renal diet. Smaller portions of lower-phosphorus seeds like hemp seeds are a better option.
4. **Large Portions of Beans and Lentils:**
   - While beans and lentils are healthy, their phosphorus content can add up quickly. Large portions should be avoided, and it's important to balance their intake with other lower-phosphorus foods.

Tips for Including Plant-Based Proteins in Your Diet

- **Portion Control:**
  - Monitor portion sizes of plant-based proteins to keep phosphorus and potassium intake within recommended limits.
- **Combine with Low-Potassium Foods:**
  - Pair plant-based proteins with low-potassium vegetables and grains to create balanced, kidney-friendly meals.
- **Preparation Techniques:**
  - Soaking beans, lentils, and certain grains can help reduce their phosphorus content, making them more suitable for a renal diet.
- **Variety:**
  - Incorporate a variety of plant-based proteins to ensure you get all essential amino acids and maintain a diverse, interesting diet.

By carefully selecting and managing plant-based proteins, individuals with kidney disease can meet their protein needs while supporting kidney health. Plant-based proteins offer a nutritious alternative to animal proteins, helping to maintain a balanced and renal-friendly diet.

4.4.3 Protein Serving Sizes

Managing protein serving sizes is crucial for individuals with kidney disease to ensure they receive adequate nutrition without overburdening their kidneys. Proper portion control helps balance protein intake, reduces waste product buildup in the blood, and minimizes strain on the kidneys.

Recommended Serving Sizes for Protein Sources

1. **Animal Proteins:**
   - **Chicken, Turkey, Fish:** A typical serving size for lean animal proteins such as chicken, turkey, or fish is about 3 ounces (85 grams), roughly the size of a deck of cards. This portion provides sufficient protein while controlling phosphorus and potassium intake.
   - **Egg Whites:** For egg whites, a serving size is typically 2 large egg whites or 1/4 cup. This portion offers high-quality protein with minimal phosphorus.
   - **Lean Pork or Beef:** When consuming lean cuts of pork or beef, a 3-ounce serving is recommended to manage protein intake without overwhelming the kidneys.
2. **Plant-Based Proteins:**
   - **Tofu:** A standard serving of tofu is about 1/2 cup or 4 ounces (113 grams). This portion provides adequate protein while being easier on the kidneys compared to animal proteins.
   - **Lentils and Beans:** For lentils and beans, a serving size is typically 1/2 cup cooked. This amount offers protein and fiber but should be monitored closely due to the phosphorus content.
   - **Quinoa:** A serving size of quinoa is about 1/2 cup cooked. Given its higher phosphorus content, it's important to keep portions small and balanced with other low-phosphorus foods.

3. **Dairy and Dairy Alternatives:**
   - **Low-Phosphorus Dairy:** For low-phosphorus dairy options, such as cream cheese or ricotta, a serving size is about 1/4 cup. Regular dairy products should be limited or substituted with kidney-friendly alternatives.
   - **Plant-Based Milks:** If using plant-based milks like almond or rice milk, a serving size is typically 1 cup. It's essential to choose unsweetened, fortified versions that are low in phosphorus and potassium.

Tips for Managing Protein Serving Sizes

- **Use Measuring Tools:**
  - Use kitchen scales, measuring cups, and portion control plates to ensure you're consuming the recommended serving sizes for proteins. This helps prevent accidental overconsumption.
- **Balance with Other Nutrients:**
  - Pair proteins with low-potassium vegetables, grains, and healthy fats to create balanced meals that support kidney health. This ensures you're not relying too heavily on protein alone for your nutritional needs.
- **Listen to Your Body:**
  - Pay attention to how your body responds to different protein portions. If you feel overly full or experience symptoms like fatigue or swelling, you may need to adjust your serving sizes.
- **Consult with a Dietitian:**
  - Work with a dietitian to personalize your protein intake based on your specific kidney function, nutritional needs, and lifestyle. They can provide tailored advice on portion sizes and meal planning.

By managing protein serving sizes carefully, individuals with kidney disease can meet their nutritional needs without overloading their kidneys. Proper portion control is key to maintaining a healthy, balanced diet that supports overall well-being and kidney function.

4.5 Dairy and Alternatives

4.5.1 Low-Phosphorus Dairy Options

For individuals with kidney disease, controlling phosphorus intake is essential to prevent complications such as bone and heart issues. Dairy products are a common source of phosphorus, so choosing low-phosphorus options is key to maintaining kidney health while still enjoying dairy in your diet.

Recommended Low-Phosphorus Dairy Options

1. **Cream Cheese:**
   - Cream cheese is a lower-phosphorus dairy option compared to harder cheeses. It can be used as a spread, in dips, or as a base for various recipes. A serving size of 1 to 2 tablespoons is typically low in phosphorus and can be included in a renal diet.
2. **Ricotta Cheese:**
   - Ricotta cheese, particularly the low-fat variety, is another lower-phosphorus cheese option. It can be used in dishes like lasagna, stuffed shells, or as a spread on toast. A 1/4 cup serving provides protein with relatively low phosphorus content.
3. **Brie and Swiss Cheese:**
   - Soft cheeses like Brie and Swiss are lower in phosphorus than many other cheeses. These cheeses can be consumed in small portions (about 1 ounce) and add flavor to a renal-friendly diet without significantly increasing phosphorus levels.
4. **Butter:**
   - While not a significant source of protein, butter is a low-phosphorus dairy product that can be used for cooking or as a spread. A small amount (1 teaspoon) adds flavor without contributing much phosphorus.

5. **Sour Cream:**
   - Sour cream, particularly in small quantities (1 to 2 tablespoons), is lower in phosphorus and can be used as a topping for dishes like baked potatoes or in recipes. Opt for low-fat versions to keep the overall fat content in check.

6. **Non-Dairy Milk (Fortified):**
   - While technically not dairy, fortified non-dairy milks like almond milk or rice milk are often lower in phosphorus than cow's milk. When choosing non-dairy milk, select unsweetened versions that are fortified with calcium and vitamin D, and low in added phosphorus.

Tips for Including Low-Phosphorus Dairy in Your Diet

- **Portion Control:**
  - Even low-phosphorus dairy options should be consumed in moderation. Stick to recommended serving sizes to manage phosphorus intake effectively.

- **Check Labels:**
  - Always check nutrition labels for phosphorus content. Some dairy products, especially processed ones, may have added phosphorus, so it's important to choose brands that are low in phosphorus.

- **Balance with Other Foods:**
  - Pair low-phosphorus dairy products with low-potassium vegetables, grains, and proteins to create balanced, kidney-friendly meals.

- **Substitute When Necessary:**
  - Consider using non-dairy alternatives or lower-phosphorus options in recipes that traditionally call for high-phosphorus dairy products. For example, use almond milk instead of cow's milk in cooking and baking.

By carefully selecting low-phosphorus dairy options and monitoring portion sizes, individuals with kidney disease can enjoy dairy products while keeping phosphorus levels in check. This helps to support kidney health and maintain a balanced, enjoyable diet.

4.5.2 Non-Dairy Alternatives

Non-dairy alternatives are valuable for individuals with kidney disease, offering options that are often lower in phosphorus and potassium compared to traditional dairy products. These alternatives can be useful for those who are lactose intolerant or seeking to reduce their phosphorus intake.

Recommended Non-Dairy Alternatives

1. **Almond Milk:**
    - Almond milk is a popular non-dairy alternative that is lower in phosphorus and potassium compared to cow's milk. Choose unsweetened varieties to avoid added sugars. Fortified almond milk provides essential nutrients like calcium and vitamin D, making it a nutritious option for those with kidney disease.
2. **Rice Milk:**
    - Rice milk is another non-dairy option that is typically low in phosphorus and potassium. Unsweetened rice milk is preferable to avoid excess sugars. It is often fortified with calcium and vitamin D, providing a nutritional boost while being gentle on the kidneys.
3. **Coconut Milk:**
    - Coconut milk, particularly the beverage variety, is lower in phosphorus and can be used in cooking or as a milk substitute. Opt for unsweetened versions and check for fortification with calcium and vitamin D. Note that coconut milk is higher in fat, so use it in moderation.
4. **Oat Milk:**
    - Oat milk is a creamy non-dairy alternative that can be lower in phosphorus than cow's milk. Look for unsweetened and fortified versions to ensure you are not consuming added sugars or excess phosphorus. It's a good option for baking and cooking as well.

5. **Hemp Milk:**
   - Hemp milk is made from hemp seeds and is generally lower in phosphorus compared to other non-dairy milks. It is also a good source of omega-3 fatty acids. Choose unsweetened, fortified hemp milk to maximize nutritional benefits while keeping phosphorus levels low.

6. **Soy Milk (in Moderation):**
   - Soy milk is a common non-dairy alternative that is higher in protein. However, it also contains moderate levels of phosphorus. It can be included in a renal diet in moderation, particularly if fortified with calcium and vitamin D.

Tips for Using Non-Dairy Alternatives

- **Choose Fortified Options:**
  - Opt for non-dairy milks that are fortified with calcium and vitamin D to help meet nutritional needs. Check the label to ensure they are low in added phosphorus and potassium.

- **Read Labels Carefully:**
  - Always review ingredient lists and nutrition labels to avoid added sugars, high levels of phosphorus, or other additives that may not be suitable for a renal diet.

- **Use in Cooking and Baking:**
  - Non-dairy milks can be used in cooking, baking, and as a beverage. They can replace cow's milk in recipes and are often suitable for making sauces, soups, and smoothies.

- **Monitor Portion Sizes:**
  - While non-dairy alternatives are generally lower in phosphorus, it's important to monitor portion sizes to manage overall nutrient intake effectively.

- **Consult with a Dietitian:**
  - Work with a dietitian to select the best non-dairy alternatives for your specific needs and to ensure they fit well with your overall dietary plan.

By incorporating non-dairy alternatives thoughtfully into your diet, you can enjoy a variety of milk-like products while managing phosphorus and potassium intake effectively. These options provide flexibility and can help maintain a balanced, kidney-friendly diet.

4.6 Fats and Oils

4.6.1 Healthy Fat Choices

Healthy fats are an important part of a balanced diet, providing essential fatty acids and helping to support overall health. For individuals with kidney disease, choosing the right types of fats is crucial to avoid excessive phosphorus and potassium intake while promoting heart health.

Recommended Healthy Fat Choices

1. **Olive Oil:**
   - Olive oil is a heart-healthy fat that is low in phosphorus and potassium. It is rich in monounsaturated fats, which can help reduce inflammation and support cardiovascular health. Use olive oil for cooking, dressings, or drizzling over vegetables and grains.
2. **Avocado:**
   - Avocado is a source of healthy monounsaturated fats and is low in phosphorus. It also provides vitamins and minerals, including potassium, but in a controlled amount. Use avocado slices in salads, spreads, or smoothies to add healthy fats to your diet.
3. **Canola Oil:**
   - Canola oil is another good option for healthy fats. It contains a balanced ratio of omega-3 and omega-6 fatty acids and is lower in phosphorus. Use it for sautéing, baking, or as a base for dressings.
4. **Flaxseed Oil:**
   - Flaxseed oil is rich in alpha-linolenic acid (ALA), an omega-3 fatty acid that supports heart health. It is low in phosphorus and can be used in salad dressings or added to smoothies. Note that flaxseed oil should not be used for high-heat cooking.

5. **Walnuts:**
    - Walnuts are a good source of omega-3 fatty acids and are lower in phosphorus compared to other nuts. They can be included in small amounts (about a small handful per serving) as a snack or added to salads and oatmeal.

6. **Chia Seeds:**
    - Chia seeds provide healthy fats and are rich in omega-3 fatty acids. They are low in phosphorus and can be added to smoothies, yogurt, or used to make chia pudding.

Tips for Incorporating Healthy Fats

- **Portion Control:**
    - While healthy fats are beneficial, they are also calorie-dense. Keep portion sizes moderate to manage overall calorie intake and prevent weight gain.

- **Use in Moderation:**
    - Balance your fat intake with other nutrients in your diet. Use healthy fats to replace saturated and trans fats rather than adding extra fats to your meals.

- **Cooking and Preparation:**
    - Choose oils with high smoke points, like canola or olive oil, for cooking. Reserve more delicate oils, like flaxseed oil, for cold applications such as salad dressings.

- **Read Labels:**
    - Be aware of the fat content in packaged foods and choose options that use healthy fats. Avoid products high in trans fats or excessive amounts of saturated fats.

- **Consult with a Dietitian:**
  - Work with a dietitian to tailor your fat choices to your specific dietary needs, ensuring you get the benefits of healthy fats while managing phosphorus and potassium levels.

By choosing healthy fats and using them appropriately, individuals with kidney disease can support heart health and overall well-being while managing their kidney health effectively. Healthy fats can enhance flavor and nutrition without compromising dietary goals.

4.6.2 Fats to Avoid

For individuals with kidney disease, certain types of fats can exacerbate health issues and complicate dietary management. Avoiding these fats helps in reducing phosphorus levels, managing cardiovascular health, and supporting overall kidney function.

Fats to Avoid

1. **Saturated Fats:**
   - **Sources:** Saturated fats are found in animal products such as fatty cuts of meat, full-fat dairy products (like cheese and butter), and certain tropical oils (such as coconut and palm oil). Processed and baked goods, including pastries and cakes, also contain high levels of saturated fats.
   - **Health Impact:** Saturated fats can increase cholesterol levels, which contributes to cardiovascular problems and can strain the kidneys. They also provide minimal nutritional benefit compared to healthier fat sources.
2. **Trans Fats:**
   - **Sources:** Trans fats are commonly found in partially hydrogenated oils used in many processed and packaged foods, such as margarine, fried foods, and baked goods (like cookies and crackers).
   - **Health Impact:** Trans fats increase bad cholesterol (LDL) levels and lower good cholesterol (HDL), leading to a higher risk of heart disease. They are also linked to inflammation and other health issues, making them harmful for individuals with kidney disease.
3. **High-Phosphorus Oils:**
   - **Sources:** Some oils, such as those used in processed snacks and fast food, may contain added phosphorus or phosphorus-based additives. Examples include certain brands of vegetable oil or margarine.
   - **Health Impact:** High-phosphorus oils can contribute to elevated phosphorus levels in the body, which can lead to complications such as bone and cardiovascular issues.

4. **Fatty Meats:**
    - **Sources:** Fatty meats, including bacon, sausage, and heavily marbled cuts of beef or pork, are high in both saturated fats and phosphorus.
    - **Health Impact:** Consuming fatty meats can lead to high cholesterol levels and increased phosphorus intake, which can strain kidney function and contribute to cardiovascular problems.
5. **Fried Foods:**
    - **Sources:** Fried foods, such as French fries, fried chicken, and doughnuts, are cooked in oils that often contain high levels of unhealthy fats and may be prepared using high-phosphorus oils.
    - **Health Impact:** Fried foods are high in trans fats and saturated fats, which can exacerbate cardiovascular issues and increase phosphorus levels, making them unsuitable for a renal diet.
6. **Cream and High-Fat Dairy Products:**
    - **Sources:** Cream, whole milk, and high-fat cheeses contain significant amounts of saturated fat and phosphorus.
    - **Health Impact:** These dairy products can contribute to high cholesterol levels and increased phosphorus intake. Choosing low-fat or lower-phosphorus dairy options is preferable.

Tips for Avoiding Harmful Fats

- **Read Labels:**
    - Check food labels for trans fats, saturated fats, and added phosphorus. Avoid products that list partially hydrogenated oils or high-fat content.
- **Choose Healthier Cooking Methods:**
    - Opt for baking, grilling, steaming, or sautéing instead of frying. These methods use less oil and can help reduce fat intake.
- **Select Lean Cuts:**
    - Choose lean cuts of meat and trim visible fat to reduce saturated fat intake. Incorporate more plant-based proteins and healthy fats into your diet.

- **Limit Processed Foods:**
  - Reduce consumption of processed and packaged foods that often contain unhealthy fats and added phosphorus. Focus on whole, unprocessed foods whenever possible.
- **Consult with a Dietitian:**
  - Work with a dietitian to tailor your fat intake and ensure that your diet supports kidney health while meeting your nutritional needs.

By avoiding harmful fats and making informed choices, individuals with kidney disease can manage their health more effectively, reduce the risk of cardiovascular issues, and maintain a balanced, kidney-friendly diet.

4.7 Beverages

4.7.1 Hydration Tips

Proper hydration is essential for maintaining kidney health and overall well-being. For individuals with kidney disease, managing fluid intake is crucial to avoid overloading the kidneys and maintaining fluid balance. Here are key hydration tips to help manage fluid intake effectively.

Hydration Tips

1. **Monitor Fluid Intake:**
   - **Guideline:** Follow your healthcare provider's recommendations on daily fluid intake. This typically includes all beverages and foods with high water content, such as soups and fruits.
   - **Strategy:** Use measuring cups or bottles to track your fluid consumption throughout the day and stay within your prescribed limits.
2. **Choose Hydrating Foods Wisely:**
   - **Options:** Incorporate foods with lower water content into your diet if fluid intake is restricted. Examples include dry grains and certain vegetables like spinach and lettuce.
   - **Avoid:** Limit or avoid high-water-content foods, such as watermelon and cucumbers, if advised to reduce fluid intake.
3. **Use Ice Chips or Small Sips:**
   - **Technique:** If you need to manage fluid intake but still want to stay hydrated, try using ice chips or taking small sips of water. This can help alleviate thirst without consuming large amounts of liquid.
4. **Opt for Low-Sodium Drinks:**
   - **Choices:** Select beverages that are low in sodium, as sodium can contribute to fluid retention and increase the burden on the kidneys.

Herbal teas and flavored water (without added sodium) can be good options.
- **Avoid:** Steer clear of sugary or high-sodium drinks like sodas and sports drinks, which can lead to increased fluid retention and other health issues.

5. **Balance with Electrolytes:**
   - **Consideration:** In cases where fluid intake is restricted, it's important to maintain a balance of electrolytes, including sodium and potassium. Electrolyte imbalances can lead to complications, so consult with your healthcare provider on appropriate sources of electrolytes.
   - **Options:** Electrolyte-balanced beverages, like certain low-sodium broths or oral rehydration solutions, can be used under medical guidance.

6. **Stay Consistent:**
   - **Routine:** Establish a consistent hydration routine based on your fluid restrictions. Consistent hydration helps maintain balance and can prevent dehydration or fluid overload.
   - **Monitor Symptoms:** Pay attention to signs of dehydration or fluid overload, such as dry mouth, dark urine, or swelling, and adjust your fluid intake accordingly.

7. **Consult with a Dietitian:**
   - **Personalized Advice:** Work with a dietitian to develop a hydration plan that meets your individual needs. They can provide tailored advice based on your kidney function, dietary restrictions, and overall health.

8. **Adjust Based on Activity:**
   - **Activity Level:** Adjust fluid intake based on physical activity levels. Increased activity may require slight adjustments in fluid intake, but always within the limits set by your healthcare provider.

Additional Considerations

- **Temperature Effects:** Be mindful of fluid intake in extreme temperatures, as hot weather can increase fluid needs while cold weather might reduce thirst. Adjust your hydration practices accordingly.
- **Medications:** Some medications can affect fluid balance, so be aware of any effects and discuss with your healthcare provider if adjustments are needed.

By following these hydration tips, individuals with kidney disease can effectively manage their fluid intake, support kidney health, and maintain overall well-being. Proper hydration management is key to balancing fluid levels and preventing complications associated with kidney disease.

4.7.2 Drinks to Limit or Avoid

For individuals with kidney disease, selecting appropriate beverages is crucial to managing fluid balance, reducing phosphorus and potassium intake, and maintaining overall health. Some drinks can contribute to excessive fluid intake, high phosphorus, or elevated potassium levels, which can complicate kidney function and overall health. Here's a guide to drinks to limit or avoid.

Drinks to Limit or Avoid

1. **Sugary Beverages:**
   - **Examples:** Sodas, sweetened teas, fruit juices, and energy drinks.
   - **Health Impact:** These drinks are often high in added sugars, which can lead to weight gain and increased risk of diabetes, exacerbating kidney issues. They may also contribute to fluid overload if consumed in large quantities.
2. **High-Sodium Drinks:**
   - **Examples:** Some sports drinks, canned or bottled soups, and vegetable juices with added salt.
   - **Health Impact:** High sodium content can cause fluid retention and increase blood pressure, putting additional strain on the kidneys. Opt for low-sodium or no-salt-added versions if necessary.
3. **High-Potassium Juices:**
   - **Examples:** Orange juice, tomato juice, and certain vegetable juices.
   - **Health Impact:** These juices are high in potassium, which can be problematic for individuals with kidney disease who need to manage potassium levels. Excessive potassium can lead to serious health issues, including heart problems.
4. **High-Phosphorus Beverages:**
   - **Examples:** Cola drinks and some energy drinks.

- **Health Impact:** Cola drinks and certain processed beverages can contain added phosphorus, which can contribute to elevated phosphorus levels in the blood. This can lead to complications like bone loss and cardiovascular problems.

5. **Alcoholic Beverages:**
   - **Examples:** Beer, wine, and spirits.
   - **Health Impact:** Alcohol can have several adverse effects on kidney health, including dehydration, increased blood pressure, and potential interactions with medications. It can also contribute to fluid overload if consumed in excess.

6. **Caffeinated Drinks:**
   - **Examples:** Coffee, strong teas, and caffeinated sodas.
   - **Health Impact:** Caffeine is a diuretic, which can increase urine output and potentially lead to dehydration. It can also impact blood pressure and kidney function, so it should be consumed in moderation.

7. **Milk (High-Phosphorus Varieties):**
   - **Examples:** Whole milk and certain types of fortified milk with high phosphorus content.
   - **Health Impact:** High-phosphorus milk options can contribute to increased phosphorus levels. Opt for lower-phosphorus milk alternatives when possible.

Tips for Managing Drink Choices

- **Read Labels:**
  - Check nutrition labels for sodium, potassium, phosphorus, and sugar content. Avoid drinks with high levels of these components to stay within dietary restrictions.

- **Choose Lower-Potassium and Lower-Phosphorus Alternatives:**
  - Opt for beverages with lower potassium and phosphorus content. Consider options like water, herbal teas, and certain non-dairy milks that fit your dietary needs.
- **Hydrate Wisely:**
  - Maintain proper hydration with beverages that are suitable for your condition. Stick to recommended fluid intake limits to avoid fluid overload.
- **Consult with a Dietitian:**
  - Work with a dietitian to determine the best beverage choices for your specific health needs. They can help you navigate drink options based on your kidney function and overall health.

By limiting or avoiding these drinks, individuals with kidney disease can better manage their health, control fluid balance, and prevent complications. Making informed beverage choices is essential for maintaining kidney function and supporting overall well-being.

4.8 Snacks and Sweets

4.8.1 Kidney-Friendly Snacks

Snacking can be part of a balanced diet for individuals with kidney disease, provided that the choices align with dietary restrictions and support overall health. Kidney-friendly snacks are those that are low in sodium, potassium, and phosphorus, and provide essential nutrients without overburdening the kidneys. Here are some healthy, kidney-friendly snack options:

Recommended Kidney-Friendly Snacks

1. **Apple Slices with Almond Butter:**
    - **Preparation:** Slice an apple and serve with a small amount of almond butter.
    - **Benefits:** Apples are low in potassium, and almond butter provides healthy fats and protein. Be mindful of portion sizes to manage phosphorus intake from nuts.
2. **Carrot Sticks with Hummus:**
    - **Preparation:** Cut raw carrots into sticks and dip them in a small serving of low-sodium hummus.
    - **Benefits:** Carrots are low in potassium and high in fiber, while hummus offers protein without excessive sodium or phosphorus.
3. **Rice Cakes with Cream Cheese:**
    - **Preparation:** Spread a thin layer of low-fat cream cheese on a rice cake.
    - **Benefits:** Rice cakes are low in potassium and phosphorus, and cream cheese adds flavor with a lower phosphorus content compared to other cheeses.
4. **Cucumber Slices with Yogurt Dip:**
    - **Preparation:** Slice cucumbers and dip them in a yogurt-based dip made from plain, low-fat yogurt.

- **Benefits:** Cucumbers are low in potassium, and plain yogurt provides protein and calcium without added phosphorus.

5. **Fresh Berries:**
   - **Preparation:** Choose berries like strawberries or blueberries and enjoy them fresh.
   - **Benefits:** Berries are lower in potassium compared to other fruits and provide antioxidants and vitamins.

6. **Popcorn:**
   - **Preparation:** Air-pop popcorn and season lightly with herbs or a pinch of salt.
   - **Benefits:** Popcorn is a whole grain and low in potassium and phosphorus. Avoid butter or excessive salt to keep it kidney-friendly.

7. **Low-Sodium Crackers with Avocado:**
   - **Preparation:** Spread a small amount of mashed avocado on low-sodium crackers.
   - **Benefits:** Avocado provides healthy fats and flavor, while low-sodium crackers are a better option for managing sodium intake.

8. **Plain Greek Yogurt with a Drizzle of Honey:**
   - **Preparation:** Enjoy plain Greek yogurt with a small amount of honey for added sweetness.
   - **Benefits:** Greek yogurt is lower in potassium and phosphorus and provides protein. Honey adds a touch of sweetness without excessive sugar.

Tips for Choosing Kidney-Friendly Snacks

- **Watch Portion Sizes:**
  - Even kidney-friendly snacks should be consumed in moderation to manage overall nutrient intake and avoid exceeding dietary restrictions.

- **Check Ingredients:**
  - Opt for snacks with minimal added sodium and avoid products with high phosphorus additives. Read labels carefully to ensure that ingredients fit within your dietary guidelines.
- **Balance Nutrients:**
  - Choose snacks that provide a balance of nutrients without compromising your kidney health. Combine protein sources with low-potassium vegetables or fruits for a satisfying and nutritious snack.
- **Consult with a Dietitian:**
  - Work with a dietitian to tailor snack choices to your specific needs. They can provide personalized recommendations based on your kidney function and overall health.

By selecting kidney-friendly snacks, individuals with kidney disease can enjoy satisfying and nutritious options while adhering to dietary restrictions. These snacks help support overall health and contribute to a balanced, kidney-friendly diet.

4.8.2 Sweets and Desserts

For individuals with kidney disease, enjoying sweets and desserts requires careful selection to ensure they fit within dietary restrictions and support overall health. When choosing or preparing sweets, it's important to consider factors such as sugar content, potassium, phosphorus, and sodium levels. Here's a guide to making kidney-friendly choices for sweets and desserts.

Recommended Kidney-Friendly Sweets and Desserts

1. **Fruit Sorbet:**
   - **Preparation:** Make sorbet from blended fruits like berries or apples with a small amount of added sweetener. Avoid high-potassium fruits such as bananas or oranges.
   - **Benefits:** Sorbet can be a refreshing treat that is lower in potassium compared to some other desserts. Use fruits that are within your dietary limits and ensure no added phosphorus or sodium.

2. **Baked Apples with Cinnamon:**
   - **Preparation:** Core an apple and bake it with a sprinkle of cinnamon. You can add a small amount of brown sugar or a drizzle of honey if desired.
   - **Benefits:** Apples are relatively low in potassium, and cinnamon adds flavor without adding sodium or phosphorus. This dessert is a warm, satisfying option.

3. **Vanilla Pudding:**
   - **Preparation:** Use a low-phosphorus, low-potassium recipe for vanilla pudding, or buy a commercial product that fits your dietary needs.
   - **Benefits:** Vanilla pudding can be a comforting dessert that is generally lower in potassium and phosphorus if made with suitable ingredients.

4. **Homemade Cookies:**
   - **Preparation:** Bake cookies using low-phosphorus, low-potassium ingredients, such as white flour and unsweetened applesauce. Control sugar content to manage overall intake.
   - **Benefits:** Homemade cookies allow you to control the ingredients and make them suitable for a kidney-friendly diet. Use recipes with minimal added sodium and phosphorus.

5. **Plain Yogurt with a Drizzle of Honey:**
   - **Preparation:** Serve plain, low-fat Greek yogurt with a small amount of honey for sweetness.
   - **Benefits:** Plain yogurt provides protein and calcium without excessive phosphorus. Honey adds a touch of natural sweetness without additional sugars.

6. **Fruit Salad:**
   - **Preparation:** Prepare a fruit salad with fruits that are low in potassium, such as apples, strawberries, and grapes. Avoid high-potassium fruits and limit added sugars.
   - **Benefits:** A fruit salad with kidney-friendly fruits offers a refreshing and nutritious dessert option. Be mindful of portion sizes and fruit choices.

7. **Angel Food Cake:**
   - **Preparation:** Make or buy angel food cake, which is typically lower in fat and phosphorus compared to other cakes. Avoid high-sodium or high-phosphorus toppings.
   - **Benefits:** Angel food cake is a light dessert that can be suitable for a renal diet when consumed in moderation. Serve with low-potassium fruit if desired.

Tips for Choosing or Making Kidney-Friendly Desserts

- **Limit Sugar Intake:**
    - Opt for desserts that use less sugar or natural sweeteners in moderation. Excessive sugar can contribute to weight gain and other health issues.
- **Watch Portion Sizes:**
    - Enjoy sweets and desserts in moderation to manage overall calorie and nutrient intake. Large portions can lead to excessive consumption of sugars and other restricted nutrients.
- **Read Labels:**
    - When buying pre-made desserts, check labels for phosphorus additives, sodium content, and sugar levels to ensure they fit within your dietary guidelines.
- **Choose Low-Potassium and Low-Phosphorus Ingredients:**
    - When baking or preparing desserts, select ingredients that are low in potassium and phosphorus. Avoid ingredients with high phosphorus content, such as certain baking powders or processed additives.
- **Consult with a Dietitian:**
    - Work with a dietitian to develop dessert options that fit your specific dietary needs. They can provide guidance on ingredient choices and portion control to align with your kidney health.

By choosing or preparing kidney-friendly sweets and desserts, individuals with kidney disease can enjoy occasional treats while adhering to dietary restrictions. These options help satisfy sweet cravings without compromising kidney health.

4.9 Condiments and Seasonings

4.9.1 Low-Sodium Options

Managing sodium intake is crucial for individuals with kidney disease to help control blood pressure and reduce fluid retention. High sodium levels can exacerbate kidney issues and lead to complications such as hypertension and swelling. Here's a guide to low-sodium options that can help you maintain a balanced diet while supporting kidney health.

Recommended Low-Sodium Options

1. **Fresh Fruits:**
    - **Examples:** Apples, berries, grapes, and peaches.
    - **Benefits:** Fresh fruits are naturally low in sodium and can provide essential vitamins and antioxidants without added salt. They are also a good source of hydration.
2. **Fresh Vegetables:**
    - **Examples:** Carrots, cucumbers, bell peppers, and spinach.
    - **Benefits:** Fresh vegetables are low in sodium and can be used in a variety of dishes. They provide important nutrients like vitamins and fiber without added salt.
3. **Lean Proteins:**
    - **Examples:** Skinless chicken breast, turkey, and fresh fish.
    - **Benefits:** Choosing fresh, unprocessed meats ensures that sodium content is minimal. Avoid processed meats like sausages or deli meats, which are often high in sodium.
4. **Low-Sodium Canned Beans:**
    - **Examples:** Low-sodium black beans, kidney beans, and chickpeas.

- **Benefits:** Look for beans labeled as "low-sodium" or "no salt added" to reduce sodium intake while still benefiting from the protein and fiber content of beans.

5. **Herbs and Spices:**
   - **Examples:** Basil, rosemary, thyme, and garlic powder.
   - **Benefits:** Using herbs and spices instead of salt can enhance the flavor of your dishes without adding sodium. Fresh herbs are especially beneficial for flavoring without increasing sodium intake.

6. **Unsalted Nuts and Seeds:**
   - **Examples:** Almonds, sunflower seeds, and chia seeds.
   - **Benefits:** Choose unsalted varieties to avoid added sodium. Nuts and seeds are good sources of healthy fats and can be a nutritious snack option.

7. **Low-Sodium Dairy Alternatives:**
   - **Examples:** Low-sodium almond milk, coconut milk, and plain low-fat yogurt.
   - **Benefits:** Opt for dairy alternatives with no added sodium. These can provide calcium and other nutrients without contributing to high sodium levels.

8. **Whole Grains:**
   - **Examples:** Brown rice, quinoa, and oats.
   - **Benefits:** Whole grains are naturally low in sodium and provide fiber, vitamins, and minerals. Choose unprocessed or minimally processed options for the best results.

9. **Homemade Soups and Broths:**
   - **Examples:** Homemade vegetable or chicken broth made without added salt.
   - **Benefits:** Making soups and broths at home allows you to control the sodium content, ensuring that they remain low-sodium and suitable for a kidney-friendly diet.

10. **Plain Water or Infused Water:**
    - **Examples:** Plain water, or water infused with slices of cucumber, lemon, or berries.
    - **Benefits:** Water is naturally free of sodium and essential for hydration. Infused water adds natural flavors without adding sodium or other additives.

Tips for Managing Sodium Intake

- **Read Labels:**
    - Always check nutrition labels for sodium content, especially in packaged or processed foods. Opt for products labeled as "low-sodium" or "no salt added."
- **Cook at Home:**
    - Preparing meals at home allows you to control the amount of salt and sodium in your food. Use herbs, spices, and salt-free seasoning blends to add flavor.
- **Avoid Processed Foods:**
    - Minimize consumption of processed and pre-packaged foods, which often contain high levels of sodium. Focus on fresh, whole foods whenever possible.
- **Use Salt Substitutes Sparingly:**
    - If using salt substitutes, check with your healthcare provider to ensure they are appropriate for your diet, as some substitutes may contain potassium or other additives.
- **Consult with a Dietitian:**
    - Work with a dietitian to develop a meal plan that meets your specific needs and helps manage sodium intake effectively. They can provide personalized advice and meal planning strategies.

By incorporating these low-sodium options into your diet, you can better manage your sodium intake and support overall kidney health. Making mindful choices helps maintain fluid balance, control blood pressure, and reduce the risk of complications associated with kidney disease.

4.9.2 Herbs and Spices

Herbs and spices are invaluable tools in a kidney-friendly diet, providing flavor and variety without adding sodium or excess calories. They can enhance the taste of meals, making it easier to adhere to dietary restrictions while avoiding processed seasonings that may contain high levels of sodium, phosphorus, or other additives. Here's a guide to herbs and spices that are beneficial for individuals with kidney disease.

Recommended Herbs and Spices

1. **Basil:**
    - **Flavor Profile:** Sweet and slightly peppery.
    - **Uses:** Great in Mediterranean dishes, salads, and sauces. Basil adds flavor without the need for added salt.
2. **Cilantro:**
    - **Flavor Profile:** Fresh and slightly citrusy.
    - **Uses:** Ideal for garnishing and flavoring Latin American and Asian dishes. Cilantro can add a burst of flavor to salsas, soups, and salads.
3. **Rosemary:**
    - **Flavor Profile:** Pine-like and aromatic.
    - **Uses:** Perfect for seasoning meats, vegetables, and potatoes. Rosemary can be used fresh or dried in a variety of dishes for added depth of flavor.
4. **Thyme:**
    - **Flavor Profile:** Earthy and slightly minty.
    - **Uses:** Works well in soups, stews, and roasted dishes. Thyme adds complexity to recipes without sodium.
5. **Parsley:**
    - **Flavor Profile:** Fresh and mildly peppery.
    - **Uses:** Commonly used as a garnish or in recipes for added freshness. Parsley also helps enhance the flavors of other herbs and spices.

6. **Garlic Powder:**
    - **Flavor Profile:** Savory and pungent.
    - **Uses:** A convenient alternative to fresh garlic, garlic powder adds a rich, savory taste to dishes. Use it in moderation to avoid overpowering other flavors.
7. **Paprika:**
    - **Flavor Profile:** Sweet and mildly smoky.
    - **Uses:** Adds color and a subtle smokiness to dishes. Paprika is excellent for seasoning meats, vegetables, and rice.
8. **Cumin:**
    - **Flavor Profile:** Warm, earthy, and slightly nutty.
    - **Uses:** Common in Indian, Middle Eastern, and Mexican cuisines. Cumin enhances the flavor of soups, stews, and spice blends.
9. **Oregano:**
    - **Flavor Profile:** Robust and slightly bitter.
    - **Uses:** Ideal for Italian dishes, pizza, and marinades. Oregano adds a bold flavor without sodium.
10. **Ginger:**
    - **Flavor Profile:** Spicy and slightly sweet.
    - **Uses:** Adds warmth and spice to both savory and sweet dishes. Fresh ginger can be used in cooking, while ground ginger works well in baking and spice blends.

Tips for Using Herbs and Spices

- **Fresh vs. Dried:**
    - Both fresh and dried herbs can be used, though dried herbs are more concentrated. Use less dried herb compared to fresh to avoid overpowering the dish.

- **Storage:**
  - Store dried herbs and spices in a cool, dark place to maintain their potency. Fresh herbs should be refrigerated and used within a week or so.
- **Experiment with Blends:**
  - Create your own salt-free spice blends to enhance flavor. Combine herbs like basil, oregano, and thyme for a versatile seasoning mix.
- **Adjust Quantities:**
  - Start with small amounts and adjust to taste. Herbs and spices can vary in potency, so it's best to taste as you go.
- **Avoid Salt-Based Seasonings:**
  - Steer clear of seasoning blends or salt substitutes that may contain high levels of sodium or potassium. Opt for pure herbs and spices.
- **Consult with a Dietitian:**
  - Work with a dietitian to ensure that your use of herbs and spices aligns with your dietary needs. They can help you create flavorful meals that fit within your nutritional guidelines.

By incorporating a variety of herbs and spices into your meals, you can enhance the flavor of your dishes without compromising kidney health. These natural flavor enhancers make it easier to adhere to a low-sodium, kidney-friendly diet while enjoying a range of delicious and satisfying foods.

Sample Menus and Meal Plans

5.1 Weekly Meal Plan

Day 1:

- **Breakfast:** Oatmeal with fresh blueberries and a sprinkle of cinnamon; Herbal tea
- **Lunch:** Grilled chicken salad with mixed greens, cucumber, cherry tomatoes, and a low-sodium vinaigrette; Whole grain roll
- **Dinner:** Baked salmon with lemon and dill; Steamed green beans; Quinoa
- **Snacks:** Apple slices with almond butter; Carrot sticks with hummus

Day 2:

- **Breakfast:** Scrambled egg whites with spinach; Whole wheat toast; Herbal tea
- **Lunch:** Turkey and veggie wrap with lettuce, bell peppers, and a whole wheat tortilla; Side salad with lemon vinaigrette
- **Dinner:** Roasted chicken breast with rosemary; Mashed cauliflower; Wild rice
- **Snacks:** Fresh pear slices; Cucumber slices with plain Greek yogurt dip

Day 3:

- **Breakfast:** Greek yogurt with a drizzle of honey and strawberries; Herbal tea
- **Lunch:** Lentil soup (low-sodium) with a side of low-sodium crackers; Mixed greens salad
- **Dinner:** Grilled tilapia with sautéed zucchini and bell peppers; Brown rice
- **Snacks:** Berries with unsalted almonds; A small apple

Day 4:

- **Breakfast:** Smoothie made with plain Greek yogurt, fresh berries, and spinach; Herbal tea
- **Lunch:** Chicken and vegetable stir-fry with low-sodium soy sauce over wild rice; Side of steamed broccoli
- **Dinner:** Baked turkey breast with roasted carrots; Whole grain roll
- **Snacks:** Sliced bell peppers with low-sodium hummus; Fresh pear

Day 5:

- **Breakfast:** Chia pudding made with unsweetened almond milk and topped with fresh strawberries; Herbal tea
- **Lunch:** Quinoa salad with cucumbers, cherry tomatoes, and lemon dressing; Side of fresh fruit (apple or pear)
- **Dinner:** Grilled shrimp with sautéed spinach and garlic; Couscous
- **Snacks:** Plain Greek yogurt with honey; Small handful of unsalted nuts

Day 6:

- **Breakfast:** Whole grain toast with avocado and a sprinkle of black pepper; Herbal tea
- **Lunch:** Tuna salad with mixed greens, cherry tomatoes, and low-sodium vinaigrette; Whole grain crackers
- **Dinner:** Baked cod with lemon and parsley; Steamed green beans; Brown rice
- **Snacks:** Fresh apple slices; Carrot sticks with hummus

Day 7:

- **Breakfast:** Egg white and vegetable frittata (spinach, bell peppers, onions); Whole wheat toast; Herbal tea
- **Lunch:** Turkey and avocado sandwich on whole wheat bread; Side of mixed greens salad with light vinaigrette

- **Dinner:** Grilled chicken breast with rosemary; Roasted Brussels sprouts; Quinoa
- **Snacks:** Fresh berries with unsalted almonds; Sliced cucumber with plain Greek yogurt dip

5.2 Exercises for kidney friendly patient

Normal active work is gainful for by and large wellbeing, including kidney wellbeing. Exercise can help manage weight, improve cardiovascular health, and control blood pressure, which is particularly important for individuals with kidney disease. However, it's essential to choose exercises that are appropriate for your health and consult with your healthcare provider before starting any new exercise regimen. Here's a guide to exercises that are generally considered safe and effective for kidney-friendly patients:

1. Low-Impact Aerobic Exercises

- **Walking:**
  - **Benefits:** Walking is a low-impact exercise that is easy on the joints and can be done at a comfortable pace. It helps improve cardiovascular health, manage weight, and enhance overall endurance.
  - **Tips:** Start with shorter walks and gradually increase the duration as tolerated. Hold back nothing 30 minutes every day, 5 times each week.
- **Cycling:**
  - **Benefits:** Stationary or outdoor cycling is a low-impact exercise that boosts cardiovascular health and can be adjusted to your fitness level.
  - **Tips:** Use a comfortable bike and start with shorter sessions. Continuously increment the time and force as your wellness gets to the next level.
- **Swimming:**
  - **Benefits:** Swimming is a full-body exercise that is delicate on the joints. It improves cardiovascular fitness, builds strength, and provides a low-impact option for those with joint issues.
  - **Tips:** Swim at a comfortable pace and use different strokes to work various muscle groups. Ensure the pool is not too cold or hot.

2. Strength Training

- **Bodyweight Exercises:**
    - **Examples:** Squats, lunges, push-ups, and leg raises.
    - **Benefits:** Bodyweight exercises help build muscle strength and endurance without requiring heavy equipment. They are effective for improving overall fitness and supporting kidney health.
    - **Tips:** Start with a few repetitions and sets, then gradually increase as your strength improves. Center around appropriate structure to forestall injury.
- **Resistance Band Exercises:**
    - **Examples:** Bicep curls, shoulder presses, and resistance band rows.
    - **Benefits:** Resistance bands provide a gentle yet effective way to build muscle strength and flexibility. They are portable and can be used for various exercises.
    - **Tips:** Choose bands with appropriate resistance levels and perform exercises slowly and with control.

3. Flexibility and Balance Exercises

- **Stretching:**
    - **Examples:** Hamstring stretch, calf stretch, and shoulder stretch.
    - **Benefits:** Stretching improves flexibility, reduces muscle tension, and enhances overall mobility. It is an important component of any exercise routine.
    - **Tips:** Perform stretches gently and hold each position for 15-30 seconds. Avoid bouncing or overstretching.
- **Yoga:**
    - **Examples:** Gentle poses such as child's pose, cat-cow stretch, and seated forward bend.
    - **Benefits:** Yoga promotes flexibility, balance, and relaxation. It can also help manage stress and improve mental well-being.

- ○ **Tips:** Choose gentle, restorative yoga classes or routines. Focus on deep breathing and listen to your body's limits.
- **Tai Chi:**
  - ○ **Benefits:** Tai Chi is a low-impact exercise that involves slow, controlled movements. It improves balance, coordination, and mental relaxation.
  - ○ **Tips:** Join a Tai Chi class or follow instructional videos. Practice consistently to encounter the full advantages.

4. Tips for Safe Exercise

- **Consult Your Healthcare Provider:**
  - ○ Before starting any new exercise program, especially if you have kidney disease or other health conditions, consult with your healthcare provider to ensure that the exercises are safe for you.
- **Monitor Your Health:**
  - ○ Focus on how your body answers work out. If you experience unusual symptoms such as dizziness, shortness of breath, or excessive fatigue, stop the activity and seek medical advice.
- **Stay Hydrated:**
  - ○ Drink plenty of water before, during, and after exercise to stay hydrated, but be mindful of fluid restrictions if prescribed by your healthcare provider.
- **Start Slowly:**
  - ○ Begin with lower intensity and shorter durations, gradually increasing as your fitness level improves. This approach helps prevent injury and allows your body to adapt to the new routine.
- **Listen to Your Body:**
  - ○ Adjust exercises based on how you feel. It's essential to keep away from overexertion and permit time for rest and recuperation.

- **Warm Up and Cool Down:**
    - Include a warm-up before starting your workout and a cool-down period afterward to prepare your body for exercise and to promote recovery.

Incorporating these kidney-friendly exercises into your routine can enhance your overall well-being, improve physical fitness, and support kidney health. Regular physical activity, combined with a balanced diet and appropriate medical care, can contribute to better management of kidney disease and overall quality of life.

Renal Diet Recipes

6.1 Breakfast

Low-Potassium Breakfast Ingredients

1. Oatmeal with Blueberries

- **Ingredients:**
    - 1/2 cup rolled oats
    - 1 cup water
    - 1/4 cup fresh blueberries
    - 1/2 teaspoon cinnamon
    - 1 teaspoon honey (optional)
- **Directions:**
    - In a small pot, bring water to a boil.
    - Add rolled oats and reduce heat to a simmer.
    - Cook for about 5 minutes, stirring occasionally, until the oats are soft and have absorbed the water.
    - Stir in the blueberries and cinnamon. Cook for an additional 1-2 minutes.
    - If desired, drizzle with honey before serving.
- **Prep Time:** 5 minutes
- **Cooking Time:** 7 minutes
- **Serving Size:** 1 bowl (about 1 cup)
- **Nutrition (Per Serving):**
    - Calories: 200
    - Protein: 5g
    - Carbohydrates: 40g
    - Fiber: 5g

- Potassium: 150mg

2. Scrambled Egg Whites with Spinach

- **Ingredients:**
  - 4 egg whites
  - 1/2 cup fresh spinach, chopped
  - 1/4 teaspoon black pepper
  - 1/2 teaspoon olive oil
- **Directions:**
  - Heat olive oil in a non-stick pan over medium heat.
  - Add chopped spinach and cook until wilted, about 2 minutes.
  - Pour in egg whites and cook, stirring gently, until scrambled and cooked through.
  - Season with black pepper.
- **Prep Time:** 5 minutes
- **Cooking Time:** 5 minutes
- **Serving Size:** 1 plate
- **Nutrition (Per Serving):**
  - Calories: 120
  - Protein: 24g
  - Carbohydrates: 2g
  - Fiber: 1g
  - Potassium: 300mg

3. Greek Yogurt with Strawberries

- **Ingredients:**
  - 1/2 cup plain Greek yogurt
  - 1/4 cup fresh strawberries, sliced
  - 1 teaspoon honey (optional)

- **Directions:**
    - Spoon Greek yogurt into a bowl.
    - Top with sliced strawberries.
    - Drizzle with honey if desired.
- **Prep Time:** 5 minutes
- **Cooking Time:** None
- **Serving Size:** 1 bowl (about 1/2 cup yogurt and 1/4 cup strawberries)
- **Nutrition (Per Serving):**
    - Calories: 130
    - Protein: 12g
    - Carbohydrates: 15g
    - Fiber: 2g
    - Potassium: 250mg

4. Whole Wheat Toast with Avocado

- **Ingredients:**
    - 1 slice whole wheat bread
    - 1/4 avocado
    - 1/4 teaspoon black pepper
    - 1/4 teaspoon garlic powder (optional)
- **Directions:**
    - Toast the whole wheat bread.
    - Mash avocado and spread it on the toasted bread.
    - Season with black pepper and garlic powder if desired.
- **Prep Time:** 5 minutes
- **Cooking Time:** 3 minutes (toasting time)
- **Serving Size:** 1 slice of toast
- **Nutrition (Per Serving):**
    - Calories: 150
    - Protein: 4g

- Carbohydrates: 20g
- Fiber: 5g
- Potassium: 250mg

5. Chia Pudding with Berries

- **Ingredients:**
    - 2 tablespoons chia seeds
    - 1/2 cup unsweetened almond milk
    - 1/4 cup fresh raspberries
    - 1 teaspoon honey (optional)
- **Directions:**
    - Mix chia seeds and almond milk in a bowl. Stir well.
    - Refrigerate for at least 2 hours or overnight until the chia seeds have absorbed the liquid and formed a pudding-like consistency.
    - Top with fresh raspberries and drizzle with honey if desired.
- **Prep Time:** 5 minutes (plus chilling time)
- **Cooking Time:** None
- **Serving Size:** 1 bowl (about 1/2 cup)
- **Nutrition (Per Serving):**
    - Calories: 180
    - Protein: 5g
    - Carbohydrates: 22g
    - Fiber: 10g
    - Potassium: 200mg

High-Potassium Breakfast Ingredients

1. Banana Smoothie

- **Ingredients:**
    - 1 medium banana
    - 1/2 cup spinach

- 1/2 cup Greek yogurt
- 1/2 cup almond milk
- 1 teaspoon honey (optional)
- **Directions:**
    - Blend banana, spinach, Greek yogurt, and almond milk until smooth.
    - Add honey if desired and blend briefly to mix.
- **Prep Time:** 5 minutes
- **Cooking Time:** None
- **Serving Size:** 1 glass (about 12 oz)
- **Nutrition (Per Serving):**
    - Calories: 250
    - Protein: 10g
    - Carbohydrates: 35g
    - Fiber: 4g
    - Potassium: 450mg

2. Avocado Toast with Tomato

- **Ingredients:**
    - 1 slice whole wheat bread
    - 1/4 avocado
    - 1/2 tomato, sliced
    - 1/4 teaspoon black pepper
- **Directions:**
    - Toast the whole wheat bread.
    - Mash avocado and spread it on the toasted bread.
    - Top with tomato slices and season with black pepper.
- **Prep Time:** 5 minutes
- **Cooking Time:** 3 minutes (toasting time)
- **Serving Size:** 1 slice of toast

- **Nutrition (Per Serving):**
  - Calories: 200
  - Protein: 4g
  - Carbohydrates: 20g
  - Fiber: 5g
  - Potassium: 400mg

3. Sweet Potato Hash

- **Ingredients:**
  - 1 medium sweet potato, peeled and diced
  - 1/2 bell pepper, diced
  - 1/4 onion, diced
  - 1 teaspoon olive oil
  - 1/4 teaspoon paprika
- **Directions:**
  - Heat olive oil in a pan over medium heat.
  - Add diced sweet potato, bell pepper, and onion. Cook, stirring occasionally, until sweet potato is tender and slightly crispy, about 15 minutes.
  - Season with paprika.
- **Prep Time:** 5 minutes
- **Cooking Time:** 15 minutes
- **Serving Size:** 1 cup
- **Nutrition (Per Serving):**
  - Calories: 200
  - Protein: 2g
  - Carbohydrates: 35g
  - Fiber: 5g
  - Potassium: 500mg

6.2 Lunch

Low-Potassium Lunch Recipes

1. Chicken and Veggie Wrap

- **Ingredients:**
    - 1 whole wheat tortilla
    - 3 oz cooked chicken breast, sliced
    - 1/4 cup shredded lettuce
    - 1/4 cup diced cucumber
    - 1/4 cup shredded carrots
    - 1 tablespoon low-fat ranch dressing
- **Directions:**
    - Lay the tortilla flat on a plate.
    - Spread the ranch dressing over the tortilla.
    - Layer the chicken, lettuce, cucumber, and carrots on top.
    - Roll up the tortilla, securing with toothpicks if needed.
    - Slice in half and serve.
- **Prep Time:** 10 minutes
- **Cooking Time:** None (using pre-cooked chicken)
- **Serving Size:** 1 wrap
- **Nutrition (Per Serving):**
    - Calories: 250
    - Protein: 20g
    - Carbohydrates: 25g
    - Fiber: 5g
    - Potassium: 300mg

2. Turkey and Apple Salad

- **Ingredients:**
    - 2 cups mixed greens
    - 3 oz sliced turkey breast
    - 1/2 apple, thinly sliced
    - 1 tablespoon sunflower seeds
    - 2 tablespoons low-fat balsamic vinaigrette
- **Directions:**
    - Arrange mixed greens on a plate.
    - Top with sliced turkey, apple, and sunflower seeds.
    - Drizzle with balsamic vinaigrette.
- **Prep Time:** 10 minutes
- **Cooking Time:** None
- **Serving Size:** 1 salad
- **Nutrition (Per Serving):**
    - Calories: 220
    - Protein: 18g
    - Carbohydrates: 15g
    - Fiber: 3g
    - Potassium: 250mg

3. Low-Sodium Tuna Salad

- **Ingredients:**
    - 1 can low-sodium tuna, drained
    - 1/4 cup plain Greek yogurt
    - 1 tablespoon Dijon mustard
    - 1/4 cup diced celery
    - 1/4 cup diced red bell pepper
    - 1 teaspoon lemon juice
    - Black pepper to taste

- ○ 4 whole grain crackers
- **Directions:**
  - ○ In a bowl, mix the tuna, Greek yogurt, mustard, celery, bell pepper, lemon juice, and black pepper.
  - ○ Serve the tuna salad with whole grain crackers.
- **Prep Time:** 10 minutes
- **Cooking Time:** None
- **Serving Size:** 1 serving (about 1 cup of tuna salad with crackers)
- **Nutrition (Per Serving):**
  - ○ Calories: 200
  - ○ Protein: 22g
  - ○ Carbohydrates: 15g
  - ○ Fiber: 3g
  - ○ Potassium: 200mg

High-Potassium Lunch Recipes

1. Quinoa and Black Bean Salad

- **Ingredients:**
  - ○ 1/2 cup cooked quinoa
  - ○ 1/2 cup black beans, drained and rinsed
  - ○ 1/4 cup diced red bell pepper
  - ○ 1/4 cup corn kernels
  - ○ 1/4 cup diced avocado
  - ○ 1 tablespoon chopped cilantro
  - ○ 2 tablespoons lime juice
  - ○ 1 tablespoon olive oil
  - ○ 1/4 teaspoon cumin
- **Directions:**
  - ○ In a large bowl, combine quinoa, black beans, bell pepper, corn, avocado, and cilantro.

- In a small bowl, whisk together lime juice, olive oil, and cumin.
- Pour the dressing over the salad and toss to combine.
- **Prep Time:** 15 minutes
- **Cooking Time:** 15 minutes (for quinoa)
- **Serving Size:** 1 bowl (about 1 1/2 cups)
- **Nutrition (Per Serving):**
  - Calories: 350
  - Protein: 10g
  - Carbohydrates: 50g
  - Fiber: 12g
  - Potassium: 700mg

2. Lentil and Sweet Potato Stew

- **Ingredients:**
  - 1 cup lentils, rinsed
  - 1 medium sweet potato, peeled and diced
  - 1/2 cup diced tomatoes
  - 1/4 cup diced carrots
  - 1/4 cup diced celery
  - 1 small onion, diced
  - 2 cloves garlic, minced
  - 4 cups low-sodium vegetable broth
  - 1 teaspoon cumin
  - 1/2 teaspoon paprika
  - 1 tablespoon olive oil
- **Directions:**
  - In a large pot, heat olive oil over medium heat. Add onion and garlic and sauté until fragrant.
  - Add sweet potato, carrots, and celery. Cook for about 5 minutes.

- ○ Add lentils, diced tomatoes, vegetable broth, cumin, and paprika. Bring to a boil.
- ○ Reduce heat and simmer for 30-35 minutes, until lentils and sweet potatoes are tender.
- **Prep Time:** 15 minutes
- **Cooking Time:** 35 minutes
- **Serving Size:** 1 bowl (about 1 1/2 cups)
- **Nutrition (Per Serving):**
  - ○ Calories: 400
  - ○ Protein: 18g
  - ○ Carbohydrates: 65g
  - ○ Fiber: 20g
  - ○ Potassium: 900mg

3. Spinach and Chickpea Salad

- **Ingredients:**
  - ○ 2 cups fresh spinach
  - ○ 1/2 cup canned chickpeas, drained and rinsed
  - ○ 1/4 cup diced red bell pepper
  - ○ 1/4 cup cherry tomatoes, halved
  - ○ 1/4 avocado, diced
  - ○ 2 tablespoons lemon juice
  - ○ 1 tablespoon olive oil
  - ○ 1/4 teaspoon black pepper
- **Directions:**
  - ○ In a large bowl, combine spinach, chickpeas, bell pepper, tomatoes, and avocado.
  - ○ In a small bowl, whisk together lemon juice, olive oil, and black pepper.
  - ○ Pour the dressing over the salad and toss to combine.
- **Prep Time:** 10 minutes

- **Cooking Time:** None
- **Serving Size:** 1 salad (about 2 cups)
- **Nutrition (Per Serving):**
    - Calories: 300
    - Protein: 10g
    - Carbohydrates: 30g
    - Fiber: 10g
    - Potassium: 650mg

6.3 Dinner

Low-Potassium Dinner Recipes

1. Grilled Salmon with Asparagus

- **Ingredients:**
    - 4 oz salmon fillet
    - 1 cup asparagus, trimmed
    - 1 tablespoon olive oil
    - 1 clove garlic, minced
    - 1 teaspoon lemon juice
    - Black pepper to taste
- **Directions:**
    - Preheat grill to medium-high heat.
    - Brush salmon and asparagus with olive oil and sprinkle with garlic and black pepper.
    - Grill salmon for 4-5 minutes per side until it flakes easily with a fork.
    - Grill asparagus for 3-4 minutes until tender.
    - Drizzle lemon juice over salmon before serving.
- **Prep Time:** 10 minutes
- **Cooking Time:** 10 minutes
- **Serving Size:** 1 plate
- **Nutrition (Per Serving):**
    - Calories: 280
    - Protein: 25g
    - Carbohydrates: 5g
    - Fiber: 2g
    - Potassium: 400mg

2. Chicken Stir-Fry with Bell Peppers

- **Ingredients:**
    - 4 oz chicken breast, sliced
    - 1/2 cup red bell pepper, sliced
    - 1/2 cup green bell pepper, sliced
    - 1/2 cup yellow bell pepper, sliced
    - 1 tablespoon low-sodium soy sauce
    - 1 tablespoon olive oil
    - 1 clove garlic, minced
    - 1/2 teaspoon ginger, grated
- **Directions:**
    - Heat olive oil in a large skillet over medium-high heat.
    - Add chicken and cook until browned and cooked through, about 5-7 minutes.
    - Add garlic and ginger, and cook for 1 minute.
    - Add bell peppers and soy sauce, and stir-fry for another 5 minutes until peppers are tender-crisp.
- **Prep Time:** 10 minutes
- **Cooking Time:** 15 minutes
- **Serving Size:** 1 plate
- **Nutrition (Per Serving):**
    - Calories: 250
    - Protein: 25g
    - Carbohydrates: 10g
    - Fiber: 3g
    - Potassium: 350mg

3. Pasta Primavera

- **Ingredients:**
    - 1 cup cooked whole wheat pasta

- 1/4 cup zucchini, diced
- 1/4 cup cherry tomatoes, halved
- 1/4 cup bell peppers, diced
- 1 tablespoon olive oil
- 1 clove garlic, minced
- 1 tablespoon Parmesan cheese, grated
- Black pepper to taste

- **Directions:**
    - Cook pasta according to package instructions and set aside.
    - In a large skillet, heat olive oil over medium heat.
    - Add garlic and cook for 1 minute until fragrant.
    - Add zucchini, tomatoes, and bell peppers, and sauté for 5-7 minutes until vegetables are tender.
    - Add cooked pasta to the skillet and toss to combine.
    - Sprinkle with Parmesan cheese and black pepper before serving.
- **Prep Time:** 10 minutes
- **Cooking Time:** 10 minutes
- **Serving Size:** 1 bowl (about 1 1/2 cups)
- **Nutrition (Per Serving):**
    - Calories: 300
    - Protein: 10g
    - Carbohydrates: 45g
    - Fiber: 8g
    - Potassium: 350mg

High-Potassium Dinner Recipes

1. Baked Sweet Potato with Black Beans

- **Ingredients:**
    - 1 medium sweet potato
    - 1/2 cup black beans, drained and rinsed

- 1/4 cup diced tomatoes
- 1 tablespoon chopped cilantro
- 1 tablespoon Greek yogurt
- 1 teaspoon lime juice

- **Directions:**
    - Preheat oven to 400°F (200°C).
    - Pierce sweet potato with a fork and bake for 45-50 minutes until tender.
    - In a small bowl, mix black beans, tomatoes, and cilantro.
    - Slice the baked sweet potato open and fill with the black bean mixture.
    - Top with Greek yogurt and lime juice.
- **Prep Time:** 10 minutes
- **Cooking Time:** 50 minutes
- **Serving Size:** 1 stuffed sweet potato
- **Nutrition (Per Serving):**
    - Calories: 350
    - Protein: 10g
    - Carbohydrates: 60g
    - Fiber: 12g
    - Potassium: 900mg

2. Lentil and Spinach Stew

- **Ingredients:**
    - 1 cup lentils, rinsed
    - 2 cups spinach
    - 1/2 cup diced carrots
    - 1/2 cup diced celery
    - 1 small onion, diced
    - 2 cloves garlic, minced
    - 4 cups low-sodium vegetable broth
    - 1 teaspoon cumin

- 1/2 teaspoon paprika
- 1 tablespoon olive oil

- **Directions:**
  - In a large pot, heat olive oil over medium heat. Add onion and garlic and sauté until fragrant.
  - Add carrots and celery, and cook for about 5 minutes.
  - Add lentils, vegetable broth, cumin, and paprika. Bring to a boil.
  - Reduce heat and simmer for 30-35 minutes, until lentils are tender.
  - Stir in spinach and cook until wilted, about 2 minutes.
- **Prep Time:** 10 minutes
- **Cooking Time:** 35 minutes
- **Serving Size:** 1 bowl (about 1 1/2 cups)
- **Nutrition (Per Serving):**
  - Calories: 400
  - Protein: 18g
  - Carbohydrates: 65g
  - Fiber: 20g
  - Potassium: 950mg

3. Quinoa Stuffed Bell Peppers

- **Ingredients:**
  - 2 bell peppers, halved and seeds removed
  - 1 cup cooked quinoa
  - 1/2 cup black beans, drained and rinsed
  - 1/4 cup corn kernels
  - 1/4 cup diced tomatoes
  - 1 tablespoon chopped cilantro
  - 1 tablespoon lime juice
  - 1 tablespoon olive oil
  - 1/2 teaspoon cumin

- **Directions:**
    - Preheat oven to 375°F (190°C).
    - In a large bowl, combine quinoa, black beans, corn, tomatoes, cilantro, lime juice, olive oil, and cumin.
    - Stuff the bell pepper halves with the quinoa mixture.
    - Place stuffed peppers in a baking dish and bake for 25-30 minutes until peppers are tender.
- **Prep Time:** 15 minutes
- **Cooking Time:** 30 minutes
- **Serving Size:** 2 stuffed bell pepper halves
- **Nutrition (Per Serving):**
    - Calories: 350
    - Protein: 12g
    - Carbohydrates: 55g
    - Fiber: 12g
    - Potassium: 800mg

6.4 Snacks

Low-Potassium Snacks

1. Apple Slices with Almond Butter

- **Ingredients:**
    - 1 medium apple, sliced
    - 2 tablespoons almond butter
- **Directions:**
    - Core and slice the apple into thin wedges.
    - Serve with almond butter on the side for dipping.
- **Prep Time:** 5 minutes
- **Cooking Time:** None
- **Serving Size:** 1 plate
- **Nutrition (Per Serving):**
    - Calories: 200
    - Protein: 4g
    - Carbohydrates: 26g
    - Fiber: 4g
    - Potassium: 220mg

2. Cucumber and Cream Cheese

- **Ingredients:**
    - 1 medium cucumber, sliced
    - 2 tablespoons low-fat cream cheese
    - Fresh dill for garnish (optional)
- **Directions:**
    - Slice the cucumber into rounds.
    - Spread a small amount of cream cheese on each cucumber slice.
    - Garnish with fresh dill if desired.

- **Prep Time:** 5 minutes
- **Cooking Time:** None
- **Serving Size:** 1 plate
- **Nutrition (Per Serving):**
    - Calories: 100
    - Protein: 2g
    - Carbohydrates: 6g
    - Fiber: 1g
    - Potassium: 150mg

3. Rice Cakes with Avocado Spread

- **Ingredients:**
    - 2 plain rice cakes
    - 1/4 avocado, mashed
    - 1 teaspoon lemon juice
    - Black pepper to taste
- **Directions:**
    - In a small bowl, mash the avocado with lemon juice and black pepper.
    - Spread the avocado mixture on the rice cakes.
- **Prep Time:** 5 minutes
- **Cooking Time:** None
- **Serving Size:** 2 rice cakes
- **Nutrition (Per Serving):**
    - Calories: 150
    - Protein: 2g
    - Carbohydrates: 25g
    - Fiber: 4g
    - Potassium: 180mg

High-Potassium Snacks

1. Banana and Peanut Butter

- **Ingredients:**
  - 1 medium banana
  - 2 tablespoons peanut butter
- **Directions:**
  - Peel and slice the banana.
  - Serve with peanut butter on the side for dipping.
- **Prep Time:** 5 minutes
- **Cooking Time:** None
- **Serving Size:** 1 plate
- **Nutrition (Per Serving):**
  - Calories: 250
  - Protein: 6g
  - Carbohydrates: 30g
  - Fiber: 4g
  - Potassium: 500mg

2. Greek Yogurt with Berries

- **Ingredients:**
  - 1 cup plain Greek yogurt
  - 1/2 cup mixed berries (strawberries, blueberries, raspberries)
  - 1 teaspoon honey (optional)
- **Directions:**
  - In a bowl, combine Greek yogurt and mixed berries.
  - Drizzle with honey if desired.
- **Prep Time:** 5 minutes
- **Cooking Time:** None
- **Serving Size:** 1 bowl

- **Nutrition (Per Serving):**
    - Calories: 200
    - Protein: 15g
    - Carbohydrates: 25g
    - Fiber: 4g
    - Potassium: 600mg

3. Sweet Potato Chips

- **Ingredients:**
    - 1 medium sweet potato, thinly sliced
    - 1 tablespoon olive oil
    - 1/2 teaspoon paprika
    - Black pepper to taste
- **Directions:**
    - Preheat the oven to 375°F (190°C).
    - In a bowl, toss sweet potato slices with olive oil, paprika, and black pepper.
    - Spread the slices in a single layer on a baking sheet.
    - Bake for 20-25 minutes, flipping halfway through, until crispy.
- **Prep Time:** 10 minutes
- **Cooking Time:** 25 minutes
- **Serving Size:** 1 plate
- **Nutrition (Per Serving):**
    - Calories: 150
    - Protein: 2g
    - Carbohydrates: 30g
    - Fiber: 4g
    - Potassium: 700mg

6.5 Desserts

Low-Potassium Desserts

1. Lemon Sorbet

- **Ingredients:**
    - 1 cup water
    - 1 cup sugar
    - 1 cup fresh lemon juice
    - 1 tablespoon lemon zest
- **Directions:**
    - In a saucepan, combine water and sugar. Heat over medium heat, stirring until sugar is dissolved. Remove from heat and let cool.
    - Stir in lemon juice and lemon zest.
    - Pour the mixture into an ice cream maker and churn according to the manufacturer's instructions.
    - Transfer to a container and freeze for at least 2 hours before serving.
- **Prep Time:** 10 minutes
- **Cooking Time:** 10 minutes
- **Serving Size:** 1/2 cup
- **Nutrition (Per Serving):**
    - Calories: 120
    - Protein: 0g
    - Carbohydrates: 30g
    - Fiber: 0g
    - Potassium: 50mg

2. Blueberry Parfait

- **Ingredients:**
    - 1/2 cup plain Greek yogurt

- 1/4 cup fresh blueberries
- 1 tablespoon honey
- 1 tablespoon granola
- **Directions:**
  - In a glass, layer half of the yogurt, blueberries, honey, and granola.
  - Repeat with the remaining ingredients.
  - Serve immediately.
- **Prep Time:** 5 minutes
- **Cooking Time:** None
- **Serving Size:** 1 parfait
- **Nutrition (Per Serving):**
  - Calories: 150
  - Protein: 8g
  - Carbohydrates: 25g
  - Fiber: 2g
  - Potassium: 150mg

3. Rice Pudding

- **Ingredients:**
  - 1/4 cup white rice
  - 1 cup water
  - 1 cup low-fat milk
  - 1/4 cup sugar
  - 1/2 teaspoon vanilla extract
  - Ground cinnamon for garnish
- **Directions:**
  - In a saucepan, combine rice and water. Bring to a boil, then reduce heat and simmer until water is absorbed, about 15 minutes.
  - Add milk and sugar to the rice, and cook over medium heat, stirring frequently, until the mixture thickens, about 20 minutes.

- Stir in vanilla extract.
- Pour into serving dishes and let cool. Garnish with a sprinkle of cinnamon before serving.

- **Prep Time:** 5 minutes
- **Cooking Time:** 35 minutes
- **Serving Size:** 1/2 cup
- **Nutrition (Per Serving):**
    - Calories: 180
    - Protein: 4g
    - Carbohydrates: 35g
    - Fiber: 0g
    - Potassium: 120mg

High-Potassium Desserts

1. Banana Bread

- **Ingredients:**
    - 2 ripe bananas, mashed
    - 1/2 cup sugar
    - 1/4 cup vegetable oil
    - 2 eggs
    - 1 cup whole wheat flour
    - 1/2 teaspoon baking soda
    - 1/2 teaspoon baking powder
    - 1/2 teaspoon cinnamon
- **Directions:**
    - Preheat oven to 350°F (175°C). Grease a loaf pan.
    - In a large bowl, combine bananas, sugar, oil, and eggs.
    - In another bowl, mix flour, baking soda, baking powder, and cinnamon.
    - Gradually add dry ingredients to wet ingredients, stirring until just combined.

- Pour batter into prepared loaf pan and bake for 45-50 minutes, until a toothpick inserted into the center comes out clean.
- **Prep Time:** 10 minutes
- **Cooking Time:** 50 minutes
- **Serving Size:** 1 slice (1/8 of loaf)
- **Nutrition (Per Serving):**
  - Calories: 200
  - Protein: 4g
  - Carbohydrates: 35g
  - Fiber: 3g
  - Potassium: 350mg

2. **Chocolate Avocado Mousse**

- **Ingredients:**
  - 2 ripe avocados, peeled and pitted
  - 1/4 cup unsweetened cocoa powder
  - 1/4 cup honey
  - 1/4 cup almond milk
  - 1 teaspoon vanilla extract
- **Directions:**
  - In a food processor, combine avocados, cocoa powder, honey, almond milk, and vanilla extract. Blend until smooth.
  - Spoon the mousse into serving dishes and refrigerate for at least 1 hour before serving.
- **Prep Time:** 10 minutes
- **Cooking Time:** None
- **Serving Size:** 1/2 cup
- **Nutrition (Per Serving):**
  - Calories: 250
  - Protein: 3g

- Carbohydrates: 30g
- Fiber: 7g
- Potassium: 500mg

3. Mango Chia Pudding

- **Ingredients:**
  - 1 ripe mango, peeled and diced
  - 1 cup almond milk
  - 1/4 cup chia seeds
  - 1 tablespoon honey
  - 1/2 teaspoon vanilla extract
- **Directions:**
  - In a blender, puree the mango with almond milk, honey, and vanilla extract.
  - Pour the mixture into a bowl and stir in chia seeds.
  - Cover and refrigerate for at least 4 hours or overnight, until thickened.
  - Stir before serving.
- **Prep Time:** 10 minutes
- **Cooking Time:** None (requires refrigeration)
- **Serving Size:** 1/2 cup
- **Nutrition (Per Serving):**
  - Calories: 200
  - Protein: 4g
  - Carbohydrates: 35g
  - Fiber: 8g
  - Potassium: 400mg

Managing Special Dietary Needs

7.1 Diabetes and Kidney Disease

Diabetes is a leading cause of chronic kidney disease (CKD), often leading to a condition called diabetic nephropathy. High blood sugar levels over time can damage the blood vessels in the kidneys, impairing their ability to filter waste and excess fluids from the blood. Managing blood sugar levels through a healthy diet, regular exercise, and medication is crucial in preventing or slowing the progression of kidney damage in individuals with diabetes. Early detection and proper management of diabetes can significantly reduce the risk of developing kidney disease.

7.2 Hypertension and Kidney Disease

Hypertension, or high blood pressure, is a major risk factor for developing chronic kidney disease (CKD). The kidneys contain numerous blood vessels, and high blood pressure can cause these vessels to narrow, weaken, or harden. This reduces blood flow, impairing the kidneys' ability to filter waste and excess fluids effectively. Over time, the damage can lead to kidney failure.

Conversely, CKD can exacerbate hypertension, creating a harmful cycle. Damaged kidneys may fail to regulate blood pressure effectively, leading to even higher blood pressure levels. Therefore, controlling hypertension is crucial for preventing kidney damage and managing CKD.

Strategies for managing hypertension and protecting kidney health include:

1. **Medication:** Antihypertensive medications help lower blood pressure and reduce the strain on the kidneys.
2. **Diet:** A kidney-friendly diet low in sodium and processed foods helps maintain healthy blood pressure levels.
3. **Lifestyle Changes:** Regular exercise, maintaining a healthy weight, limiting alcohol intake, and avoiding smoking are essential for managing hypertension and protecting kidney function.

Early detection and management of hypertension are critical to preventing or slowing the progression of kidney disease. Regular check-ups and monitoring of blood pressure and kidney function can help individuals at risk maintain their health and avoid complications.

7.3 Vegetarian/Vegan Renal Diet

Following a vegetarian or vegan diet while managing kidney disease can be challenging but entirely feasible with careful planning. A plant-based renal diet focuses on selecting foods that support kidney health while providing necessary nutrients without overloading the kidneys.

Key Considerations:

1. **Protein Sources:** While animal proteins are restricted, plant-based proteins from sources like tofu, tempeh, lentils, and beans can be included in moderation. However, because legumes and some nuts and seeds are high in potassium and phosphorus, portion control is essential.
2. **Potassium Management:** Many fruits and vegetables are rich in potassium, which needs to be monitored closely. Opt for low-potassium options such as apples, berries, carrots, and cauliflower, and limit high-potassium foods like bananas, potatoes, and avocados.
3. **Phosphorus Control:** Phosphorus is found in many plant foods, including whole grains, nuts, seeds, and certain vegetables. Using phosphorus binders as prescribed by a healthcare provider and choosing lower-phosphorus options, such as white rice, refined grains, and some vegetables, can help manage phosphorus levels.
4. **Calcium and Vitamin D:** Since dairy products are typically restricted in a renal diet, ensure adequate calcium and vitamin D intake through fortified plant-based milks, leafy greens, and supplements if necessary.
5. **Sodium Limitation:** Processed plant-based foods can be high in sodium. Focus on whole foods and prepare meals at home to control salt intake, using herbs and spices for flavor instead.
6. **Fluid Intake:** Monitor fluid intake as prescribed by your healthcare provider, especially if there is a risk of fluid retention.

Sample Meals:

- **Breakfast:** Oatmeal made with water or almond milk, topped with blueberries and a sprinkle of flaxseeds.
- **Lunch:** Mixed green salad with cucumbers, bell peppers, and a tahini dressing, served with a side of quinoa.
- **Dinner:** Stir-fried tofu with low-potassium vegetables like green beans and red bell peppers, served with white rice.
- **Snacks:** Apple slices with almond butter or rice cakes with avocado spread.

Benefits:

A vegetarian or vegan renal diet can provide numerous health benefits, including improved blood pressure control, better blood sugar management, and reduced inflammation. It also supports overall health and well-being by encouraging the consumption of nutrient-dense, fiber-rich foods.

Consultation:

Working with a registered dietitian specializing in renal nutrition can help tailor a vegetarian or vegan diet to meet individual nutritional needs and ensure it supports kidney health. Regular monitoring of kidney function, potassium, phosphorus, and other nutrient levels is crucial to maintaining a balanced and effective diet.

Living with a Renal Diet

8.1 Dining Out Tips

Dining out while managing kidney disease can be enjoyable with some careful planning and smart choices. Here are a few tips to help you navigate restaurant menus:

1. **Research Ahead:** Look up the restaurant's menu online before going out. Many places provide nutritional information, allowing you to identify kidney-friendly options in advance.
2. **Ask Questions:** Make sure to your server about how dishes are ready. Request modifications such as reducing or omitting salt, choosing grilled instead of fried items, and substituting high-potassium sides with lower-potassium options.
3. **Portion Control:** Restaurant servings are often larger than recommended portions. Consider sharing a meal with a friend, or ask for a to-go box to save half for later.
4. **Choose Wisely:** Opt for grilled or baked proteins, and select low-potassium vegetables. Avoid creamy sauces and dressings, which can be high in sodium and phosphorus.
5. **Hydration:** Monitor your fluid intake, especially if you're on a fluid restriction. Avoid high-sodium beverages like sodas and opt for water or unsweetened tea.

With these strategies, you can enjoy dining out while keeping your kidney health in check.

8.2 Traveling with a Renal Diet

Traveling with a renal diet requires a bit of extra planning, but it's entirely manageable. Here are a few hints to assist you with remaining focused:

1. **Pack Snacks:** Bring along kidney-friendly snacks such as unsalted nuts, rice cakes, fresh fruits like apples and berries, or pre-cut low-potassium vegetables like cucumbers and carrots.
2. **Research Destinations:** Look up restaurants and grocery stores at your destination that offer renal-friendly options. Many places currently give nourishing data on the web.
3. **Stay Hydrated:** Carry a reusable water bottle and be mindful of your fluid intake. Avoid high-sodium beverages like sodas and choose water or unsweetened tea.
4. **Plan Ahead:** If staying in a hotel, book a room with a kitchenette. This allows you to prepare your own meals and control ingredients.
5. **Communicate Needs:** Inform airlines, hotels, and restaurants of your dietary requirements ahead of time to ensure suitable meal options are available.

By preparing in advance, you can enjoy your travels without compromising your kidney health.

8.3 Coping with Dietary Changes

Adapting to dietary changes for kidney health can be challenging but manageable with the right approach. Here are a few strategies to help:

1. **Educate Yourself:** Understand the dietary restrictions and why they are necessary. Knowledge can help you make informed choices and stay motivated.
2. **Plan and Prepare:** Create meal plans and prep meals in advance. This reduces stress and ensures you always have kidney-friendly options available.
3. **Seek Support:** Connect with a dietitian or join support groups to share experiences and get practical advice.
4. **Focus on Taste:** Experiment with herbs and spices to enhance flavor without adding sodium. Discover new recipes to keep meals enjoyable.
5. **Be Patient:** Adjusting to dietary changes takes time. Give yourself grace and stay positive as you transition to a new eating routine.

These steps can help ease the adjustment and make the dietary changes more manageable and sustainable.